CINEMATIC PROPHYLAXIS

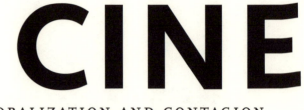

CINE

GLOBALIZATION AND CONTAGION

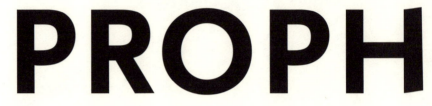

PROPH

DUKE UNIVERSITY PRESS

DURHAM AND LONDON

2005

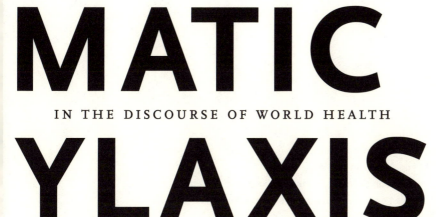

MATIC

IN THE DISCOURSE OF WORLD HEALTH

YLAXIS

KIRSTEN OSTHERR

© 2005 Duke University Press
All rights reserved
Printed in the United States of America on acid-free paper ♾
Designed by *Andrew Shurtz*
Typeset in Scala and Scala Sans by Tseng Information Systems, Inc.
Library of Congress Cataloging-in-Publication Data
appear on the last printed page of this book.

The case, to the writer, therefore, appears something like this: As a nation we believe in high standards of living. We believe in sanitation, in pure food, in pure milk, in the best obtainable hygiene, instruction, and education for our children. Is it possible that the color and content of their minds is a matter of indifference to us? We pay for our school system. We pay for our water supply. We also pay for the motion pictures. What would we say if any questionable character were to be allowed to come in suddenly and take charge of our children's schooling? Or, if suspected water were even occasionally turned into our mains? What an outcry goes up if a milk supply in a town is suddenly discovered to be in the least degree tainted! The vast haphazard, promiscuous, so frequently ill-chosen, output of pictures to which we expose our children's minds for influence and imprint, is not this at least of equal importance? For, as we cannot but conclude, if unwatched, it is extremely likely to create a haphazard, promiscuous and undesirable national consciousness.

HENRY JAMES FORMAN, *Our Movie Made Children*

Contents

Illustrations

Acknowledgments

Research and writing can often feel like solitary activities, but the end product bears traces of the many friends, colleagues, family members, archivists, and librarians who have enabled this project to come to fruition. The time has come to thank them, formally.

Although I could undoubtedly go back further, my thanks begin with three influential professors who encouraged me and shaped my thinking while I was an undergraduate at Reed College: Jacqueline Dirks, Christine Mueller, and Jaume Martí-Olivella. Those wonderful, formative years would not have been as fruitful without them.

In graduate school at Brown University, where this project first took shape, I found challenging and rewarding intellectual provocation from my dissertation director, Mary Ann Doane, and from my other readers, Mari Jo Buhle and Phil Rosen. Film research during those years wouldn't have been nearly as much fun without the encyclopedic brain and twisted humor of Richard Manning, film archivist extraordinaire. I shared many seminars, reading and writing groups, and film outings with my cherished friends in grad school, but perhaps more importantly, we also shared many wonderful meals and reminded each other when it was time to stop talking (and thinking) about work. For their intellectual camaraderie and friendship I thank Kirsten Lentz, Karl Schoonover, Rosalind Galt, Jonna Eagle, Charlotte Biltekoff, Natasha Zaretsky, and Kristin Sollenberger.

The challenges of the research undertaken for this book were made easier by the skill and generosity of many experienced hands: The Staff of the History of Medicine Division at the National Library of Medicine and the staff of the Moving Images and Sound Branch of the National Archives were immensely knowledgeable and helpful during my many research trips to those archives. The members of the Interlibrary Loan office at the Sciences Library at Brown University tirelessly tracked down almost-out-of-print 16 mm films and videos, aiding immeasurably in my research. More recently, the Interlibrary Loan staff of Fondren Library at Rice University has also been exceptionally helpful. In addition to these professional contributions, funding from the Office of the Dean of Humanities at Rice University has been vital to the final completion of this book.

My thanks also go to Ken Wissoker at Duke University Press for his enthusiasm for this project and to Anitra Grisales and the rest of the tremendously helpful staff at Duke Press. Special thanks also go to Lisa Cartwright and Melani McAlister for their careful readings of the manuscript, their insights and interest, and their willingness to serve as mentors from afar.

Portions of this manuscript were published previously as articles. Chapter 2 originally appeared as "Contagion and the Boundaries of the Visible: The Cinema of World Health" in *Camera Obscura* 50, no. 17 (2002): 1–39. Part of chapter 3 was published as " 'Invisible Invaders': The Global Body in Public Health Films" in Les Friedman, ed., *Cultural Sutures: Medicine and Media* (Duke University Press, 2004).

Finally, the oldest and deepest thanks go to my family. They have always been a great source of support, encouragement, and perspective. My aunts Trisha and Kathy and my uncle Jim have been sources of good cheer and have reminded me to get my nose out of the books once in a while. The memories of my grandparents, my father Fritz, and my aunt Margy have in varied ways fueled my curiosity about and passion for excavating little known aspects of the past. Extra special thanks go to my mother Mary Ellen and my sister Gretchen, who have been truly inspirational in their own lives and great cheerleaders for mine. They helped me keep my eyes on the prize. And my last, most tender thanks go to PVK, who has made this ending a joyful new beginning.

Cinema and Hygiene

From World War Two and the Korean conflict health education prospered
as the physical and mental defectiveness of the nation was revealed.

RICHARD K. MEANS, *A History of Health Education in the United States*

VISIBLE SYMPTOMS AND TECHNOLOGIES OF REPRESENTATION

Recent attempts to halt the spread of severe acute respiratory syndrome
(SARS) in China (in 2003) and foot-and-mouth disease in western Europe
(in 2001) have been undermined by the invisibility of contagion. Spread
by airborne viruses capable of surviving transcontinental travel, these outbreaks have prompted widespread efforts to fortify local and global boundaries against the flow of disease. The increasing prevalence of infectious
disease pandemics has provoked extensive commentary on both the impossibility of maintaining national boundaries in the era of globalization and
on the medieval insularity of the quarantine measures enacted against contaminated regions. This contrast between postmodern global interconnect-
edness and premodern isolationism highlights the extent to which the ever-
expanding culture of surveillance faces a unique representational challenge
in the realm of public health. Despite the adoption of painstaking strategies
for eliminating diseases by eliminating infected animals and quarantining
infected people, efforts to halt the flow of contagion have been frustrated by
the difficulty of visually representing the virus. While images of slaughtered
animals, face masks, and decontamination procedures at airports have filled
the media coverage of these epidemics, the impossibility of ascertaining the
precise location of the virus until after the fact makes the threat of a new
outbreak seem ever present.

In many ways, the discourses of globalization and invisible contagion surrounding these recent outbreaks are on a continuum with the depictions of disease outbreaks in post–World War Two public health films. In both cases, invisible pathogens produce widespread anxieties about global contagion, and in both cases, the anxiety is displaced through a proliferation of images of contamination.[1] This form of representational inoculation—if one can see the contaminant, one can avoid infection—defines the discourse of world health, with its efforts to map and thereby contain disease-ridden areas of the globe. This discourse compulsively attempts to visually represent invisible contagions in order to fix the location of the ever-elusive pathogen. In both postwar and contemporary representations of the spread of contagion, the search for images of disease fetishizes the invisible interior of the human body—where the contagious "difference" may be hidden—as the site of a privileged form of knowledge. The intersections of the invisible global flow of contaminated objects and the invisible contagion lurking within the human body form the focus of this project.

Cinematic Prophylaxis is an interdisciplinary study of public health and Hollywood films that represent the spread of contagious disease across national borders. In the broadest sense, the book argues that a discourse of world health develops and becomes increasingly culturally pervasive from World War Two to the present day. Audiovisual materials play a crucial role in the articulation of world health, not only as vehicles of educational and ideological dissemination, but also as metaphors for the spread of disease within the processes of globalization. The communications technologies— such as film, television, and satellites—that enabled multilingual, international instruction in the postwar era by the Centers for Disease Control and the World Health Organization were widely celebrated as media that could facilitate the globalization of culture and promotion of world health. But the content of these films reveals a contradictory attitude toward the dissolution of national boundaries that takes place in the era of globalization. Even while postwar public health films embrace the ideals of world health on one level, they simultaneously invoke a distinct and deeply anxious mode of representing the spread of contagious disease across national borders.

This anxiety shares with recent outbreaks the concern with realism in representations of invisible contagion. In both cases, it is crucial that the visualization of disease bear an indexical relation to the object itself, so that "authentic" documentary images of contagion can function as inoculations against the continued spread of disease.[2] Cinema's privileged relationship to indexicality is claimed in a wide range of discourses, with varying ideological effects. This has been an ongoing issue from the invention of photography to the present postphotographic digital era, and the ability to distinguish fiction from reality in visual representations has been a central problem for the cinema of public health. With its aim of training entire nations of viewers to imagine the presence of invisible pathogens in scenarios of consumption and exchange, the project of world health is confronted with the simultaneous need for indexical evidence of the presence of disease and for artificial simulations of the spatial and temporal flow of contagion through networks of social interchange.

The demand for convincing images of contagion has resulted from the genuine and pressing need to find effective strategies for responding to infectious disease outbreaks. Often, such responses are generated in emergency situations that require immediate action and, consequently, foreclose the possibility of time-consuming reflection upon the best means of communicating health information to the general public. At such moments, the explanation and depiction of contagion tends to fall back on familiar and, therefore, easily comprehensible imaging techniques. While the desire to prevent disease and promote health undeniably serves the greater good, the means by which this end is achieved have had unintended and sometimes quite damaging consequences. The dependence upon historically entrenched images and narratives to convey information about disease has encouraged the ongoing stigmatization and neglect of certain social groups and geographical regions, whose collective health and well-being has suffered as a result. For this reason, historical perspective on the techniques employed in the promotion of public health—especially the default mechanisms invoked at crisis moments—is of vital importance. As *Cinematic Prophylaxis* demonstrates, many of the presently familiar health education techniques have their origins in the founding moments of "world health," after World War Two. But this history involves both continuity and change, and the formative and transitional phases of this discourse provide a crucial perspective on the processes by which certain representational strategies become longstanding iconographies of disease, while others are discarded as they become outdated. The following example will illustrate this point, as the film under discussion typifies an early-twentieth-century approach to health education and points to the transformations in the representation of contagion that would occur in the postwar period.

HOW DISEASE IS SPREAD

Between 1922 and 1924, a film series called *The Science of Life* was coproduced by the U.S. Public Health Service and a small, independent production company called Bray Studios.[3] The series consists of twelve short films ranging in topics from *The Fly as a Disease Carrier* to *Personal Hygiene for Girls* and *First Aid Treatment after Exposure to Syphilis*. Many of the films in the series emphasize how proper diet and exercise will enable healthy physical and mental development and lead to good marriages producing "well-born" children. With its goal of promoting healthful living, this collection of short films typifies the rhetoric of early educational health films.

One of the particularly intriguing films in the series, *How Disease Is Spread*, begins with a sequence of intertitles explaining the viewer's civic responsibility to prevent the spread of contagious disease:

> Do you know that about one and one half MILLIONS of deaths occur every year in the United States? Do you know that over THIRTY PER CENT of this number of deaths could be PREVENTED? The remedy for this appalling condition lies in each one of us knowing how disease is transmitted and DOING HIS SHARE TO PREVENT THE TRANSMISSION. The traveler in the next scene is suffering from tuberculosis. She will show you how disease carriers may sow the seeds of a dangerous malady.[4]

The film follows the diseased traveler through a day of shopping and dining out with friends and, using a rudimentary special effect, marks the woman's path of destruction with stars left on the sites of contagion. We see the protagonist carelessly spread her germs across town as she engages in various acts of leisurely consumption, beginning with her arrival onscreen in a taxicab. Before paying her fare, the contaminated woman coughs into a handkerchief, which she replaces in her purse next to the cash that she hands to the driver. The scene alternates between medium and close-up shots, always

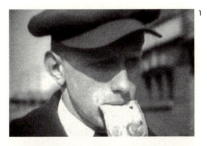

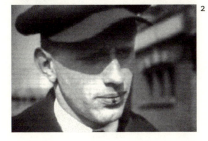

How Disease Is Spread (1924)

privileging the moment of contagion with a cut-in, so that when the cabby sticks the bill in his mouth as he digs for change in his pocket, the impropriety of this act is emphatically stated to the audience (figure 1). Once the transaction has been completed, we see another close-up of the driver's mouth, this time with a black star on his lip (figure 2).

In the next sequence, the tubercular woman strolls up to a newsstand and begins browsing through a magazine; an intertitle informs the viewer of the potential danger in such an activity: "Suppose that she has the habit of moistening her fingers when turning the pages of books." The woman coughs into her hand, and is left with stars on her fingers. The medium shots of the protagonist flipping the pages are intercut with close-ups as she licks her starred thumb and then leaves a star on the corner of each page that she turns. Shortly, the woman tires of this magazine, tosses it aside, picks up another, buys it, and walks offscreen. As the woman exits, a man enters from the opposite side of the frame and picks up the contaminated magazine. He, too, licks his thumb before turning each page and thus the stars on the page corners are transferred to his lip.

The repetition within this film of the female protagonist's contagious interventions into public life is symptomatic of the eugenicist ideological program of the series as a whole. A foundational premise of the eugenics movement is the insistence upon proper breeding, with the attendant requirement that procreative men and women pursue pure lifestyles that will produce strong and healthy babies. For women, adherence to the conventional gender norms of domestic femininity is axiomatic, and the consequences of departing from the norm are shown clearly in *How Disease Is Spread*; the extroverted woman infects a male consumer through her inappropriate behavior at the newsstand, and in the next sequence, she infects an innocent youth, potentially destroying the child's future mating capabilities.

In both of these scenes, the sphere of contagion is not only the public sphere but also, importantly, the sphere of commercialized leisure. While *How Disease Is Spread* attempts to specify the process by which invisible germs move from person to person, it also unwittingly links the process to particular scenarios that only occur in modern, urbanized consumer culture. The commodification of activities such as transportation, communication, and food service creates a circuit of exchange that enables diseases to spread through networks of production and consumption. It is no accident that in each of these scenes contagion occurs through the exchange of money; the cinematic representation of the body enables a commodification of the human form, both onscreen and in the paying audience, and the process of transforming individual identity into a consumable object becomes interwoven with the process of contagion in this period, as the public sphere becomes a site of both entertainment and contamination.[5]

In the next scene, the woman enters a restaurant and is seated with another woman and a young girl (presumably mother and daughter). The intertitle ominously sets the stage: "If we could see the bacteria on a drinking glass which has been used by a disease-carrier." After the woman takes a sip of water, the camera cuts in to a point-of-view close-up of the rim of the glass, covered with stars. In a medium shot of the table, we see the little girl asking her mother for water, and when her glass appears empty, the "disease-carrier" offers her own glass. As the girl drinks from the contaminated vessel, the intertitle informs us, "This shows why certain articles used by different persons should be sterilized." When we return to the lunch scene, the girl has a star on her lip.

The use of the close-up in this film is significant not only as a technique for displaying the presence of germs, but also as a mode of fragmenting and fetishizing the human body. By using this representational technique, *How Disease Is Spread* reveals an early expression of the discourse of contagion, which places great emphasis on the importance of maintaining coherent, nonfragmented organic and national bodies, despite its inability to represent such bodies as whole.[6] Thus, even this early public health film contains the contradiction that comes to define the postwar discourse of contagion, which seeks to visually represent that which is invisible, just as the fetish—here, the commodity fetish—stands for something that is not actually there.[7] While the stars can signify the paths of contagion to the viewer, the characters in the film cannot see them. Thus, the film is attempting to train viewers to imagine seeing germs that they cannot actually see. *Imagining* the presence of disease is crucial to the construction of the public sphere in the discourse of public health; viewers are trained to identify scenarios of contagion, but in the process of categorizing threatening situations, these films also categorize threatening characters, threatening social types.

In *How Disease Is Spread*, the threatening character is the middle-class white woman, whose participation in the public sphere is seen as contaminating. The linkage of middle-class white women with contamination in this film would seem to contradict their traditional social status as guardians of the private sphere who must be protected from the dangers of the public sphere.[8] Indeed, in one of the more prevalent early-twentieth-century discourses of modernity, the public sphere was characterized as a dirty, crowded, and alienated mass of industrial workers, whose anonymity enabled criminality to pass undetected. The true sources of immorality were obscured by the thronging crowds of the new urban centers, and consequently all but the most sanctioned participants in the public sphere (namely, the normative white, propertied, literate males) were subject to suspicious scrutiny. In this vision of modernity, the middle-class white woman is representative of the domestic sphere and serves as the antidote to the evils of the public sphere—but only if she stays at home. Thus, while most discourses of modernity linked the typology of the diseased character with racial or class difference, the eugenicist perspective of *How Disease Is Spread* expanded the definition of disease carriers to include misbehaving middle-class white women as problematic subjects of modernity. Despite the continued and widespread rhetorical linkage of whiteness and femininity with purity, the discourse of contagion promoted near-universal suspicion as an unfortunate but necessary precaution. Therefore, public health films were produced to assist good citizens in imagining, based on a brief glance, what lurked within their fellow city dwellers, to determine whether they were corrupt or legitimate participants in the public sphere.

How Disease Is Spread thus sought to fulfill, for an early-twentieth-century audience, one of the same functions that photography had fulfilled starting in the previous century. Allan Sekula argued in his account of the intersection of technologies of representation and scientific discourses of racial and moral purity:

> In claiming to provide a means for distinguishing the stigmata of vice from the shining marks of virtue, physiognomy and phrenology offered an essential hermeneutic service to a world of fleeting and often anonymous market transactions. Here was a method for quickly assessing the character of strangers in the dangerous and congested spaces of the nineteenth-century city. Here was a gauge of the intentions and capabilities of the other.[9]

And indeed, in many discourses of modernity, the typology of the diseased character was linked with racial or class difference from the norm of middle-class whiteness. However, in this widely viewed public health film, the good character has turned evil. Not only has she spread disease to the cab driver, the magazine reader, and her fellow diner, but, as the film goes on to illustrate, "By such careless habits, one diseased individual may scatter infection across an entire continent." Following this proclamation, the viewer is presented with an animated map of the United States containing a superimposed list of infectious diseases: "Gonorrhea, Syphilis, Diphtheria, Smallpox, Tuberculosis, Measles, Influenza, Scarlet Fever, Common Colds, etc." As this list fades out, a new caption appears: "Carrier of an Infectious Disease," located near a dot on the map in the Northeast United States, which is identified by a pointer. The map dissolves and is replaced by a closer view of the dot in the Northeast region, where more dots appear, with the caption "Infections from the Disease Carrier." As the pointer taps each new infection, another caption explains, "Each infected person becomes in turn the

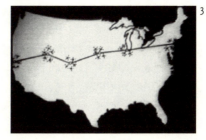

source of further infections," and new "secondary infection" rings appear. At this point the film cuts back to the full map of the United States, and a line traces the path of contagion across the country, connecting the dots, leaving new rings of secondary infections, and finally linking the coasts with the trail of disease (figure 3).[10]

This film's selection of the least likely candidate for representing social contamination was undoubtedly strategic, as the emphasis on lifestyle—the infected woman's "careless habits"—was a key component of the rhetoric of consumerism during this period, and advertisements for personal hygiene products were directed primarily toward middle-class white women.[11] The discourse of consumerism played a key role in defining the public sphere as urban space was transformed by technological and cultural developments such as the automobile, the department store, and the expansion of nickelodeons and vaudeville stages into motion picture palaces. These developments not only created a sphere of commercialized leisure, they also offered women increased opportunities to participate in the public sphere without requiring a male companion or chaperone.[12] As part of this transformation, the development of mass communication technologies enabled education of the audience in techniques for preventing the spread of contagions as well as mass indoctrination into an epistemology linking disease with the public sphere's "dirty masses." Ironically, this mass-mediated discourse constructed as its ideal audience an imagined community[13] of innocent, healthy people whose boundaries are defined by their racial, national, and class "purity" (as long as they behave properly, as our protagonist did not), and yet the audience's very presence in the public space of a motion picture theater in 1924 would implicate them as members of the public that they were being instructed to avoid.[14]

By approaching public health practice as an issue of lifestyle, *How Disease Is Spread* represents the prevention of contagion as a responsibility of the individual, not the community. While this film recognizes contagion as a national problem, it does not place disease in the context of globalization or world health and, therefore, does not emphasize the problem of maintaining national borders as an extension of the physical boundaries of the self. This emphasis on local rather than global outbreaks links the representation of contagion to a gendered conception of domestic consumer culture, in contrast to the sexual and racial transnational public sphere that will define the postwar period. Instead of linking contagion to sexualized physical border crossing or racialized national border crossing, the representation of contagion here is closely tied to gender—the purveyor of contagion in this film is a white, middle-class woman whose pathological status is tied to her unhealthy forms of consumerism. In *How Disease Is Spread*, the paths of contagion are equated with paths of consumption, particularly in the context of commercialized leisure. But popular culture is not perceived as a global phenomenon until after World War Two, and thus the representation of the sphere of consumption remains within u.s. borders in this film.[15] In contrast, later public health films directly emphasize the importance of the national border as a site of surveillance and bodily regulation. Despite the fact that international quarantine is a crucial component of the practice of public health from at least the eighteenth century onward, the cinematic representation of contagion is not linked with the global flow of bodies until after World War Two.

While analysis of a single film cannot provide sufficient evidence of the dominant modes of representation in an entire historical period, viewed in the context of other early health films, the *Science of Life* series as a whole offers a useful contrast with later films, if largely through negative definition. That is, the earlier films are most notable for what they lack, in comparison with postwar public health education. Formally and stylistically, the *Science of Life* series exemplifies early public health filmmaking before the decisive shift to sound in the late 1920s—the use of voiceover in postwar films is a crucial strategy for identifying aurally what the films cannot successfully depict visually.[16] Thematically, the series demonstrates this period's tendency to understand health through the dual frames of modern, gendered consumer culture and the eugenicist ideology of racial and sexual purity. These themes become inseparable in postwar films, as questions of health and hygiene become inextricably linked to issues of globalization.

A PARTIAL HISTORY OF CONTAGIOUS CINEMA

The history of public health film production is linked to the history of early cinema through their mutual construction of—and by—the broader surveillant impulse of late-nineteenth- and early-twentieth-century modernity, with its emphasis on the regulation of individual and national bodies. Motion pictures and institutions of public health were reshaping the public sphere in this period, with the aim of preventing a range of moral and biological contagions. Although very little government-sponsored public health filmmaking took place between *The Science of Life* series (1922–24) and the u.s. entry into World War Two, the realms of educational and commercial production and exhibition were not as separate in that period as they are today.[17] In the postwar period, health films were isolated from all other forms of cinematic entertainment, and yet, simultaneously, they came to occupy a central location in the public imagination of national identity. The events leading up to this seemingly contradictory state of affairs are the focus of chapter 1.

Using *How Disease Is Spread* (1924) as a point of reference for my discussion of postwar public health films will elucidate the historical specificity of the scope and vectors of contagion that distinguishes pre– and post–World War Two films. While communication and commerce (including the trade in motion pictures) had been global long before World War Two, the concept of "globalization" only gains audiovisual discursive prominence after the war. Through a cinematic emphasis on transnational air travel, communications technologies, and cartographic representations of the global flow of bodies and objects, cinematic articulations of the spread of disease expand their boundaries from the national to the global after 1945. Linked to this development is a shift in the modes of visualizing invisible contagions. A dialectic of visibility and invisibility pervades the imagery of contagion throughout its history, but specific socially legible markers of disease displace contagion from gender deviance, in the films of the 1920s, to racial and sexual transgression in the postwar films. These categories are not mutually exclusive but, rather, have varying degrees of visible salience in different representational paradigms. Thus, the gender improprieties of the female disease carrier in the earlier film are implicitly linked to eugenicist discourses of racial and sexual "purity," but the specific techniques of visualization in that film emphasize gender over race and sexuality.

In all of the film analyses that follow, my privileging of particular categories of difference is driven by the historically specific context in which the film was produced and viewed. This context consists of generic and thematic groupings of films, iconographic linkages across genres, popular and scientific discourses about cinema and public health, and broader cultural concerns articulated across different media. Since my argument is both medium-specific and more broadly historical, motion pictures provide the central set of "documents," but my textual analysis is governed by the films' relationship to contemporaneous treatises about the role of cinema in public life. These treatises, in turn, are informed by the social, political, and cultural milieu in which they (and the films) were produced and consumed. For instance, a postwar public health film like *The Fight Against the Communicable Diseases* (1950) is considered in relation to other postwar public health films, public health issues and policies, and public health discourses about the role of motion pictures in promoting and disseminating the ideology of world health. Simultaneously, however, the film is viewed in relation to popular motion pictures of the period that also engage with questions of the invisible spread of contagious disease, such as science fiction alien invasion films. Finally, the widely discussed social issues of Communism and civil rights are considered in relation to the intersecting imagery of alien or viral invasion of national and bodily boundaries.

While the various intertextual histories of cinema and public health provide a crucial framework for analyzing the significance of these films, certain types of historical evidence are regrettably absent from this study. I have not included written records pertaining to the production, distribution, and exhibition of these films, because they are largely nonexistent or, at best, scattered across the country in unofficial collections unknown to researchers. No comprehensive history of public health film production exists, and consequently, much of the research for this project involved the challenging—if seemingly basic—task of simply identifying and locating copies of relevant films.[18] While several archival collections of historical audiovisual materials do exist, most do not contain documentation about the films, nor do they claim to be comprehensive in any sense. Although there is abundant evidence to suggest that these films were far from obscure or marginal, they were nonetheless treated as ephemeral objects; possessing neither the artistic nor the commercial value deemed necessary to merit preservation, the films and the records related to them were often discarded as the age of video made the medium of 16 mm film obsolete.[19]

Thus, the central task of this project was to develop an understanding of the range and variety of health films that were produced throughout the twentieth century, especially after World War Two, in order to identify repeated themes and modes of representation. It is certainly possible that focused research on a single film might yield fruitful information about who made the film, where it was shown, who saw it, and what they thought of it; it is equally possible that such a search might lead only to a dead end. So, despite my curiosity about these important details, I made the strategic decision to focus here on text and context, leaving production and reception for another project. This methodology raises the question of how legitimately to interpret a film with only partial access to the historical materials that might provide a more complete answer. In other words, it raises the question of how to determine when one might be "reading too much into" a given film. And yet, having access to information about the film's producers would not necessarily help answer this question—an auteur's best executed intentions for a film cannot guarantee that the message will be received.[20] For that matter, having access to the audience members' responses to a film would not necessarily prove that the film "meant" what they said it meant, either.[21] Moreover, as film scholar Ruth Vasey has shown, the regulation of Hollywood film under the Production Code was specifically designed to produce a degree of textual ambiguity that not only enabled but in fact encouraged viewers to "read into" the obfuscations and innuendo that defined popular film in this period.[22] By approaching these films as collective evidence of a broader discursive formation, I have attempted to identify widespread cultural concerns that the films were expressing—whether consciously and intentionally or not. In other words, my interpretation of these films was guided by my identification of specific issues and concepts that were repeated frequently enough to convince me that they functioned as "common sense" in a wide range of materials related to the promotion of postwar public health in the United States and abroad.

In the first chapter, I trace the intersection between public health organizations and institutions of motion picture reform. More specifically, this chapter examines the development of the educational public health film in relation to debates over the social and artistic role of cinema in the public sphere of the 1930s. The proliferation of treatises on the "entertainment" versus "educational" value of film in this period ultimately led to the reinforcement of the Hollywood Production Code in 1934, and the language of these debates was heavily influenced by the discourse of contagion. Health education films were linked with instruction and opposed to films associated with pleasure, and yet the official articulation of boundaries between these spheres of discursive production could not keep them apart. Instead, the dominant representational forms of world health came to define the representation of a wide range of contagions in popular culture in the postwar period.

The interconnections between educational and entertainment films are especially striking considering the intense institutional pressure to isolate each mode of representation from the other. But this is not merely a formal or stylistic point; on the contrary, the efforts to create "realistic" visual representations of the invisible bind the most didactic instructional films with the most spectacular fictional features. Collectively, these films constitute the audiovisual discourse of world health, and the appearance of consistent, cross-generic techniques for visualizing contagion strongly suggests that the ideals of world health thoroughly pervaded both scientific and popular cultures in the postwar period. Moreover, the widespread dispersion of this imagery helps to account for its historical durability; as we can see in the foot-and-mouth and SARS epidemics, in the language of computer viruses, and in popular film and television, the rhetoric of contagious globalization continues to appear in prominent mass-mediated cultural forms.

Following my discussion of the "education versus entertainment" debates, I examine the status of film as a technology of ideological and instructional reproduction within global health surveillance organizations, arguing that although film was a privileged medium of discourse for these institutions, it was also identified as a source of the very contagions that public health organizations were meant to contain. Chapter 2 provides the historical context for the surveillant gaze and the discourse of contagion by examining some key moments of institutional and representational intersection in the histories of public health and cinema: the "bacteriological revolution" of the 1880s, the invention of cinema in the 1890s, the Spanish American War in 1898, and World Wars One and Two. At each of these moments, the technologies of monitoring and visually representing contagious disease become increasingly systematic in their modes of production. By tracing this history, I demonstrate that the parallels between public health and cinematic institutionalization and representation emerge from historical forces engaged with the fear of invisible contagions. Moreover, I argue that the same anxiety that drives health surveillance organizations in their frustrated attempts to represent contagious disease is reproduced in the organizations' privileging of film as the medium whose unique ability to capture "the real" will enable the elusive invisible to be visualized. As I demonstrate in my analysis of two postwar public health films—*Hemolytic Streptococcus Control*, a 1945 U.S. Navy training film, and *The Eternal Fight*, a 1948 United Nations film—a dialectic of visibility and invisibility pervades the films that attempt to represent contagious disease. The tension within these films, between indexical representation of the body and the impossibility of visualizing potential threats to that body's integrity, reveals the paranoia about maintaining organic national boundaries that underlies the supposed confidence of the globally hegemonic postwar United States.

After examining the attempts to separate public health and Hollywood modes of representation in chapter 1 and discussing the techniques for representing invisible disease invasions in chapter 2, the third chapter argues that this institutionalized regulation is circumvented through the different film genres' shared participation in broader discourses of visuality and disease. By comparing postwar public health films and postwar science fiction films, I demonstrate that the dialectic of visibility and invisibility at the heart of the pursuit of world health also structures the central problematic in an important subgenre of 1950s cinema: the alien invasion narrative. In these films, the oscillation between indexical and artificial representations of the invisible shifts to an oscillation between stock footage and special effects, enacting the same anxiety to visually fix the location of contagion.

A key argument of chapter 3 is that the prevailing interpretation of post-war science fiction invasion films as "Communist allegories" fails to recognize a crucial element common to all of the films: the centrality of the body in representations of invasion and contagion. The dialectic of visibility and invisibility is crucial to films such as *Invasion of the Body Snatchers*, as well as to the public health films discussed in chapter 2, because these films are fundamentally preoccupied with the question of how to discern visible evidence of the interior corporeal truth of an individual. Here, instead of determining whether an individual is healthy or diseased, the problem is determining whether an individual is human or alien. In both cases, the threatened penetration of physical and national boundaries links the representational form to the globalization anxiety of world health.

The popularity of the genre of science fiction in the 1950s is crucially linked to the expansion of image-based culture in the postwar era; the proliferation of electronic images and sounds in this period is attended by an increasingly widespread expression of the compulsion to visually represent invisible contagions. In the fourth chapter, I examine the narrative structure that organizes this "compulsion" in both public health and Hollywood films: the structure of conspiracy. As discussed in earlier chapters, at the core of the dialectic of visibility and invisibility are competing versions of realism, which alternately rely on "indexical" images of racially and sexually marked bodies and "artificial" animated maps of contagion. This contradictory but nonetheless foundational drive toward realism positions both public health and Hollywood films in an anxious relationship to "the real": the impossibility of capturing a profilmic image of contagion is figured as the impossibility of mapping the boundaries of a global conspiracy. And the "crisis of referentiality" often attributed to postmodern systems of signification extends not only to the paradigmatic representational form of this era—the narrative of conspiracy—but also to the ambiguously indexical technique of epidemiological cartography.

Chapter 4 links the conspiracies of alien invasion in science fiction films of the 1950s with the conspiracies of globalized transportation and communication networks that enable the transnational spread of invisible contagions. By tracing this mode of representation through an important conspiracy film of the 1970s—*The Andromeda Strain*—chapter 5 explores the collapse of sexually and racially marked bodies with "alien" vectors of contagious disease. In this and earlier alien conspiracy films, the representation of globalization as both cause and cure of contagion produces a paranoia about boundary crossing that treats male bodily invasion as sexual penetration. Thus, anxieties about the spread of disease are often represented through a fear of "homosexual contagion"—a fear that takes on increased political potency in the era of AIDS (acquired immunodeficiency syndrome). Chapter 5 examines the broader shifts in the discourse of contagious globalization by analyzing AIDS education videos as texts that reveal key representational and political struggles in the transformation from the era of conspiracy to the digital era. The most recent articulations of the ideals of world health come together in the 1995 Hollywood film *Outbreak*, through a condensation of AIDS allegories and digital imaging technologies. Unlike the earlier attempts to visualize invisible contagions, digital manipulations of the filmed image in *Outbreak* seamlessly integrate the indexical and the artificial, thus fulfilling the world health desire to incorporate global surveillance technologies within the physical body. But simultaneously, the advent of digital technologies has prompted a recycling of the rhetoric of viral invasion and contagious globalization.

The recurring themes of globalization, contagion, racial and sexual difference, and technologies of representation are brought up to date in the book's conclusion through a brief discussion of computer viruses. In charting the articulation of the ideals of world health in these various genres, *Cinematic Prophylaxis* illustrates the historical transformation of national and bodily boundary anxieties from extraterrestrial to geopolitical borders between "inner" and "outer" space. Moving from early cinema in chapter 1 to contemporary cultural forms in the final section, the conclusion argues that film's supposedly privileged access to "the real" has continually failed to secure an indexical image of contagion, resulting not in discursive failure but, rather, in a proliferation of attempts to visualize the invisible.

CHAPTER I

Public Sphere as Petri Dish;

OR, "SPECIAL CASE STUDIES OF MOTION PICTURE THEATERS WHICH ARE KNOWN OR SUSPECTED TO BE FOCI OF MORAL INFECTION"

"A movie a week" is with us a national slogan, almost a physical
trait absorbed by the children with their mother's milk.

HENRY JAMES FORMAN, *Our Movie Made Children*

PLEASURE AND INSTRUCTION

In the early twenty-first century, a typical trip to the movies almost anywhere
in the United States involves driving to a megaplex and watching a Hollywood blockbuster. The chances of seeing a nonfiction film at such a theater
are minimal, with occasional noteworthy exceptions.[1] At this point in history, specific film genres are so closely tied to specific screening venues that
the arrangement seems unremarkable (to the extent that it is even recognized). However, this situation did not arise organically out of the natural development of the film industry. On the contrary, the separation of fiction and
nonfiction film exhibition was the result of strategic regulatory mechanisms
designed to protect motion pictures from censorship (that is, to protect the
profits of the Hollywood studios).

While neither the studio system nor the Production Code remains in
effect today, the vestiges of content regulation are still with us in the form
of the ratings system. The idea that a governing body might oversee the
distribution of movies to theaters and restrict access to certain types of
films thus seems familiar and again, unremarkable. Through the notion of
age-appropriate content, the Motion Picture Association of America (MPAA)
stratifies the audience according to a system that allows viewers progres-
sively increased access to graphic depictions of sex and violence over time. Although this system might provide a legitimate rationale for preventing nine-

year-olds from viewing excessively "mature" content, it does not explain why educational films that have nothing to do with sex or violence are also essentially prohibited from mainstream commercial theaters. One obvious explanation might be that the film industry is a business like any other, and educational films simply do not make money. Another explanation might be that audiences go to the movies to be entertained, and nonfiction films are too serious, pedagogical, or otherwise demanding to be much fun to watch. And yet, until the 1930s, fiction and nonfiction films were exhibited side by side, in the same theaters, often on the same bill. Clearly, then, the prevailing wisdom on what kinds of films make money and what constitutes entertainment has changed over time. A major goal of this chapter is to explain how and why these changes took the shape they did.

But even as fiction and nonfiction film venues have obviously been separated, the boundaries between these categories of film are anything but clearly defined. This might seem paradoxical given the ease of identifying the lone documentary film among the blockbusters when it does make its rare appearance at the local megaplex. However, as many film scholars have noted, fictional films have long depended on the same kinds of realism that endow documentaries with their sense of authenticity, while documentaries, in turn, have always borrowed narrative and other techniques from fiction film genres. In other words, although the exhibition practices associated with educational and entertainment films would seem to imply that these are very different types of films requiring utterly distinct viewing environments, a comparison of their respective modes of representation would suggest the opposite conclusion. This is especially true of the set of films I will be discussing in this book—the films that collectively form the discourse of world health. This archive of films consists of both instructional public health films and Hollywood feature films, and the efforts to separate the two types of films are as interesting and revealing as the degree of overlap in their representational techniques.

Consider the case of *Prevention of the Introduction of Diseases from Abroad* (1946), and *Panic in the Streets* (1950).[2] *Prevention* is a public health film, *Panic* is a Hollywood film, but both address the invasion of the United States by invisible and deadly contagious diseases hidden within the bodies of immigrants. The history of public health is punctuated by cases of specific nationalities being ostracized as vectors of ethnic ailments, especially in the period of mass immigration to the United States from 1880 to 1924.[3] While certain objective markers of difference, such as language, might easily distinguish ethnic identity, cultural stereotyping often relied more heavily on abstracted forms of visually perceptible signs, and this was especially true in the medium of film. While *Prevention* is an instructional documentary and *Panic* is an entertaining fiction, the modes of representing invisible contagions in these films are strikingly similar, despite their production well after the Production Code officially separated education and entertainment in 1934.

In *Panic in the Streets*, contagious disease enters the United States through the body of an illegal Eastern European immigrant who is shot to death on his first night in the country as retribution for leaving a card game on a winning streak. An autopsy reveals that the man would have died of pneumonic plague anyway, and thus begins a frantic race against time to locate the person who shot the immigrant as well as anyone else who may have had contact with the disease carrier. Since the plague is spread through airborne pathogens, the possibility of mass contamination is great, as is the need for identification and containment of infected persons. Thus, one of the central narrative tensions of the film is set up: how to conduct a search for contagious individuals whose symptoms will be internal and, therefore, invisible, until it is too late to cure them or trace their contacts. Added to the problem of detecting disease carriers is the problem of containment; the search must be conducted secretly in order to prevent public panic and mass evacuation of the city, which could lead to the spread of plague throughout the country. As in many public health films of the period, *Panic in the Streets* solves the problem of invisible contagions through a visual collapse of bodily signifiers of ethnicity and disease.

The search for carriers of plague thus becomes a search for external markers of internal conditions, and those markers initially take the form of a taste for ethnic cuisine—specifically, shish kebab—as the central clue to the location of potential contacts with the original carrier of plague. The conflation of the signifiers of ethnicity with the signifiers of disease pervades the discourse of world health, with its visual association of disease and permeable national and organic bodily boundaries. In this film, the consumption

4 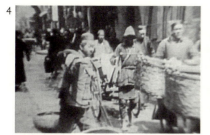 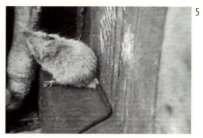 5

6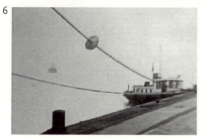

Prevention of the Introduction of
Diseases from Abroad (1946)

of ethnic food literalizes the feared border crossing from outside to inside the body, and the embarrassed admission of fondness for this exotic food by a "nonethnic" USPHS officer in *Panic in the Streets* confirms the paranoia that structures the world of international health regulation.

While both films narrate the pursuit of contagion by the USPHS, *Prevention of the Introduction of Diseases from Abroad* explains in great detail the techniques for stopping invisible contagions from crossing national borders. Accompanied by a booming, authoritative voiceover, the film consists of documentary footage of immigrants disembarking on Ellis Island and submitting to visual investigation by the camera and the USPHS officers. The status of the onscreen bodies as potentially diseased "others" is narrated through reference to global epidemiological maps that trace the spatial and temporal flow of contagion through a series of displacements. For instance, text from *Webster on Pestilence* appears onscreen, explaining that, "This disease is constantly present in the Orient, and this fact makes it an ever-present threat to the United States and its possessions." Following this proclamation, documentary images of purportedly diseased bodies in that locale appear onscreen (figure 4). The scene then cuts abruptly to a close-up of a rat, while the voiceover observes, "The germ that causes bubonic plague is carried by fleas that live on rats and other rodents. Rats are great travelers, and vessels at port must use rat guards to keep them from coming aboard" (figures 5 and 6). The metonymic slippage from disease to "Oriental" bodies to rats performs the racialized anxiety about invasion of national and bodily boundaries by invisible contagions that permeates the discourse of world health.[4] Moreover, this sequence encapsulates the film's conception of globalization as the process by which foreign diseases gain entry into the United States— a perspective shared by *Panic in the Streets.*

The assumption that plague did not exist in the United States until it arrived on a ship carrying foreign seamen clearly identifies global transportation as a primary vector of invasion and contagion. This linkage is explicitly recognized in public health policy, literature, and films, where it is often noted that the modernization of transportation technologies has been attended by an expansion in the scope of communicable diseases.[5] This recognition is often depicted cinematically through epidemiological maps, and in both *Panic in the Streets* and *Prevention of the Introduction of Diseases from Abroad,* the imagined lines of movement across the globe posit transportation itself as a conspiratorial agent linked with the contaminating invasion of national borders that inevitably accompanies the process of globalization.

The threat posed by transnational mobility is articulated in *Panic in the Streets* when the USPHS officer (Dr. Reed) demands that the local newspaper refrain from printing a story on the potential outbreak of plague. The character fears that such an announcement might provoke the widespread "panic" of the film's title, followed by a mass exodus from the infected city, and "anyone who leaves town endangers the entire country." When the mayor resists this logic, understanding the problem as specific to the local community, Dr. Reed asks him if he thinks he's living in the Middle Ages, arguing that, "Anybody that leaves here can be in any city in the country within ten hours. I could leave here today and I could be in Africa tomorrow. And whatever disease I had would go right with me!" By implicitly recognizing the concept of world health, this monologue encapsulates the centrality of disease to the film's understanding of the relationship between the local and the global. Here, interstate and international transportation are themselves understood as threats to public health which can be curtailed only by enforcing immobility on a population contained within closely regulated borders.

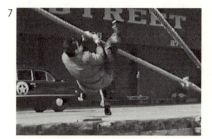

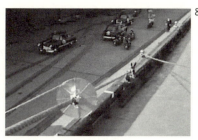

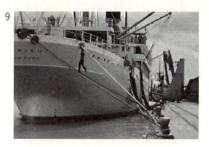

Panic in the Streets (1950)

As we see in the climactic sequence of *Panic in the Streets*, the regulation of national boundaries against penetration by invisible contagions takes a form uncannily similar to the sequence from *Prevention of the Introduction of Diseases from Abroad* described above. The "ethnic" criminal who murdered the original carrier of plague is infected himself, and at the end of the film both the police and the USPHS pursue him in the shipyards of New Orleans. In a desperate attempt at escape, the criminal scales a rope anchoring an outbound vessel to the wharf, but he is foiled, like the rodent in *Prevention*, by a simple rat barrier (figures 7–9). While viewers of *Panic in the Streets* may not necessarily have seen *Prevention of the Introduction of Diseases from Abroad*, there is an assumed audience comprehension of the purpose of the device on the rope, which functions not only to provide narrative closure (the criminal and disease carrier is caught; the rat is prevented from escaping national borders), but also to consolidate a tropic relationship that develops throughout both films between immigration, disease, and criminality. Based on such visual relationships, we can see that the representation of alien and viral invasion—in both educational and entertainment films—is integrally linked to conceptions of nation and globalization within the discourse of world health.

This brief comparison illustrates one of many cases in which the attempted separation of public health and Hollywood modes of representation is circumvented through the different films' shared participation in broader discourses of visuality and disease. As we will see, the rhetoric of contagion pervades the debates about motion picture regulation in the 1930s, but the consignment of medical and health-related themes to the realm of nonfiction educational cinema failed to eliminate the preoccupation with invisible contagions from pictures designated for entertainment purposes only. But why were these film genres separated in the first place?

SPECTATORSHIP AS CONTAGION

While films like *Prevention of the Introduction of Diseases from Abroad* and the earlier *How Disease Is Spread* (1924) might seem to be motivated by the fairly straightforward and innocuous goal of health education, such films were in fact subject to a great deal of scrutiny, criticism, and, ultimately, censorship. The u.s. government's entry into film production during World War One had persuaded numerous voluntary and commercial organizations of cinema's propagandistic capacities, and after the war, many attempted their own public education campaigns.[6] But as moving images increasingly permeated every aspect of daily life in the United States, reformers became more adamant about the need for standardized regulation of cinema's potentially harmful effects. At the same time that government health surveillance organizations became involved with health film production, the exhibition of health-related motion pictures for entertainment in commercial theaters came under attack.

Debates abounded over the social and artistic role of cinema in the public sphere of the 1930s, and the discourse arising out of these debates was centrally concerned with the intersections of spectatorship and contagion (both moral and biological). The proliferation of treatises on the "educational" versus "entertainment" value of film in this period formed the context for the policy debates that ultimately resulted in the stricter and more heavily enforced content regulation of the Hollywood Production Code in 1934. Because they were seen as excessively realistic, educational films—especially health education films—became casualties of the institutionalized separation of pleasure and instruction that resulted from the revision of the Production Code.

This redefinition of theatrical entertainment effectively functioned as a public quarantine of educational films by restricting their exhibition to noncommercial venues, and this division left the production of health films largely in the hands of government organizations.[7] But cuts in public health funding after World War One and the economic depression of the 1930s severely limited both noncommercial and government public health filmmaking between World Wars One and Two; by 1934 the realm of commercial health film production was also severely circumscribed.[8] However, despite minimal production of purely educational health films in this period, the years between the end of Hollywood's silent film production in the late 1920s and the beginning of systematic enforcement of the Production Code in 1934 allowed for cinematic experimentation with a variety of topics — including health and medicine — that would later be eliminated from the major studios' repertoires. The films produced during these years, and the debates about how they should be regulated, defined the context for the postwar development of the discourse of world health.

In order to understand the role of public health films in shaping American popular culture after World War Two, we must first examine the diverse uses of film in public education as well as the fears about the medium's potential as an educational tool that galvanized reform movements to regulate the content and exhibition of motion pictures in the 1930s. While public schools employed motion pictures only sporadically in this period, early-twentieth-century health departments utilized an ever-expanding variety of media, including motion pictures, to distribute public health information. In their role as public educators, municipal health departments helped construct the discourse of contagion by rhetorically linking a citizen's health with his or her public identity. As John Duffy has demonstrated, from the very beginnings of institutionalized public health, some form of mass media — broadsides, pamphlets, or newspapers — always fulfilled the crucial function of informing the public about techniques for avoiding contagions. During the 1880s the audience for these publications expanded from health professionals to the general public, and school health programs became an important venue for education as well.[9] Motion pictures on health were a natural extension of this tradition of mass-mediated dissemination of health information.

The efforts of school reformers were part of a larger social concern for the health of children—a concern linked to an emerging view of the public sphere as both "melting pot" and oversized petri dish. Since the development of bacteriology, the domain of disease surveillance had greatly expanded, redefining the spaces of public and private life as spheres of contagion. The public school was an ideal site of surveillance, not only because the close proximity of the students to each other created optimum conditions for contagion, but also because, as state-regulated institutions, the schools could function as sites of prevention through education, inspection, and vaccination of children. Although schools did not extensively employ audiovisual technologies of instruction until after World War Two, a small but significant number of films were shown in public schools between World Wars One and Two, including the *Science of Life* series (1922–24).[10]

By participating in the regulation of immigrant behavior, the schools provided an important context for early health film exhibition. Once immigrants had passed the Public Health Service's inspection at the nation's borders, they were subjected to a variety of Progressive reform initiatives, such as in-school training in domestic science, aimed at assimilating the newcomers into American cultural and social institutions.[11] Since attendance was compulsory, schools could reach more immigrants than the settlement houses and other reform movements that shared the mission of teaching health and hygiene as a means of "Americanizing" foreigners. Motion pictures played a key role in this reeducation, starting in the early twentieth century. Viewed by reformers as both positive and negative influences on newcomers' understanding of what it meant to be American, motion pictures were alternately celebrated and decried for their perceived influence over the purportedly simple-minded audiences of women, immigrants, and children, who were seen as incapable of easily distinguishing the moving images from reality.[12] The influence of motion pictures as mass purveyors of cultural values was recognized as early as 1907, when movies were first censored for fear of their detrimental influences on vulnerable viewers. And yet, in this same period, social reformers were attempting to marshal the medium for their own campaigns by producing pictures and organizing screenings of films that they considered to be morally uplifting.[13]

The transition to synchronized sound contributed in large part to the formal adoption and reinforcement of the Production Code in 1934, but both of these events were significantly influenced by the social scientific reform environment of the time. In 1927, the first all-sound feature, *The Jazz Singer*, was produced by Warner Brothers at a cost of $500,000.[14] The film grossed $2.5 million, and its success alerted moral reformers to the sudden expansion of the possible "evils" of the motion pictures, whose new expressive abilities seemed to suggest the industry's increasing cultural and economic power.[15] The enormous cost of the transition to sound, which rapidly became a prerequisite to economic viability in the highly competitive film industry, hit during the peak years of the Depression, when motion picture audiences were dwindling as impoverished Americans opted for the cheaper new form of entertainment offered by radio. This combination of factors drove large numbers of theaters and film production companies out of business and made the cost of production prohibitive for the marginally lucrative public health film industry.[16] Under these circumstances, the demand for minimal expenditure and maximal profitability was even greater than usual, and one result was the concentration of production in genres with broad audience appeal. Not surprisingly, the popular taste tended not to coincide with the elevated standards of the antivice reformers.

Debates about the role of motion pictures in maintaining the boundaries of public decency brought a wide range of film genres under scrutiny. Hollywood studio features, "exploitation" quickies, and educational films alike were all potential sites of discursive production about the spread of contagious disease, but the wide range of representational forms available to a viewer of such films was perceived by the reform-minded as confusing at best and morally contaminating at worst. Prior to the reinforcement of the Production Code in 1934, all of these different types of films could be viewed at the same theater, even on the same bill, and by a widely heterogeneous audience. This unregulated output of images led film reformers to debate the appropriate boundaries of different representational forms: what types of films should be seen by what types of audiences, under what circumstances, and to what effect? The coming of sound and the revision of the Production Code produced the occasion for extensive public debates over the consequences of cinematic realism for the national culture. The extent to which this debate was framed through the rhetoric of public health and hygiene reveals how central notions of contagion were to the commonsense understanding of the threat posed by nationwide distribution of unregulated mass media—a concern that only intensified when the sphere of circulation was explicitly recognized as global after World War Two.

While certain popular genres received a great deal of attention from anti-vice reformers, especially gangster films and gold digger films, other less critically noted genres also flourished during this period. These films—the vice film, the expeditionary film, and the racial adventure film—depended for their narrative incitement upon a logic of purity and contamination that exploited the trope of border crossing as simultaneously life threatening and irresistibly tantalizing. Drawing as they did on the popular fascination with hygiene, these films also share a mode of representation that pervades later public health films: they treat the bodies of sexually and racially marked "others" as exotic discoveries to be examined, regulated, and socially controlled. This pre-Code concern with the boundaries of the physical body later becomes a preoccupation with the boundaries of the national body under assault by invisible contagions. Films about venereal disease, exotic journeys, and racial fantasies share the predilection for pseudo-documentary, pseudo-scientific examinations of "exotic" races from faraway lands that later characterizes the cinema of world health. For pre-Code Hollywood, secrets of untold pleasures (such as uninhibited sexuality) and horrors (such as cannibalism) are hidden within "premodern" bodies, while in public health films they hide the source of contagions that will threaten the civilized world, if permitted to cross the imaginary international boundaries of modernity.[17]

Because of Hollywood's institutionalized emphasis on vice and because the talkies could convey more explicit suggestions of impropriety than silent films—through racy dialogue, double entendres, and so forth—the technological development of synchronized sound raised the ire of moral reformers and social scientists alike, leading to endless tirades about the effects of motion pictures on various vulnerable audiences, most notably the nation's immigrant youth.[18] Significantly, the language of motion picture reform in this period borrowed heavily from the discourse of public health. Thomas

Doherty describes the historical context that gave rise to the motion picture reform movement of the early 1930s: "For progressive reformers and cultural conservatives who beheld in the embryonic medium the potential for social damage and moral blight, the products of the motion picture industry (no less than the methods of meat packing or the distribution of demon rum) warranted regulation and prohibition as a public health measure."[19]

A nationwide network of health surveillance was established when state departments of public health achieved uniformity during the 1930s. At the same time, the systematic regulation of motion picture content by the revised and reinforced Production Code of 1934 established a nationally uniform system of representation. The standardized regulation of both of these fields in the early 1930s points to an important parallel: both institutions were reshaping the public sphere with the aim of preventing the spread of bacterial, moral, and ethnic contagions (via film spectatorship or urban squalor), and both were dedicated to the "Americanization" of immigrants through their hygienic efforts.[20]

Until the early 1930s, the opponents of Hollywood had consisted primarily of Protestant ministers and women's organizations who claimed, as self-appointed guardians of public morality, that Hollywood was directly responsible for many of the dramatic changes that had taken place in American society since the motion picture was invented. Alarmed at an increasing divorce rate, a rise in juvenile delinquency, and what they saw as a general flaunting of traditional values by American youth, the reformers blamed the movies for the nation's moral collapse. The ministers and women's organizations considered themselves "experts" on obscenity, claiming that, although they could not define it, they knew it when they saw it.[21] And in the case of the movies, anything they saw on the screen that offended their sense of propriety, whether it was social, political, or moral in nature, was defined as obscene and deserved to be banned.[22] The Production Code and its supporters wanted Hollywood's films to emphasize that "the church, the government, and the family were the cornerstones of an orderly society and that success and happiness resulted from respecting and working in this system."[23] They believed that entertainment films, because of their powerful and widespread influence, had a duty to "reinforce religious teachings that deviant behavior, whether criminal or sexual, costs violators the love and comforts of home, the intimacy of family, the solace of religion, and the protection of law. In short, they believed films should be twentieth-century morality plays that illustrated proper behavior to the masses."[24]

As Father Daniel A. Lord (a Jesuit priest and author of the 1930 Production Code) viewed Hollywood's responsibility, films were first and foremost "entertainment for the multitudes" and as such carried a "special Moral Responsibility" requisite of no other medium of entertainment or communication.[25] Unlike the audience self-selectivity of books, plays, and newspapers, the universal popularity of the movies cut across social, political, and economic classes and penetrated communities from the most sophisticated to the most remote. From Lord's perspective, the universality of the movies meant that filmmakers could not be permitted the same freedom of expression allowed to the other media of communication.[26] Movies had to be more restricted, because the picture palaces and the beautiful, glamorous stars combined to create an "ultimate fantasy" that was more persuasively and indiscriminately seductive than the illusions produced by other media. In 1928, when synchronized sound was added to the striking visual images, a sensation was created that film reform advocates believed would be "irresistible to the impressionable minds of children, the uneducated, the immature, and the unsophisticated."[27] In fact, children and uneducated laborers did represent a large percentage of the national film audience, and because this massive demographic was believed to be incapable of distinguishing between fantasy and reality, industry self-regulation or external control was deemed necessary. The Production Code of 1930 advocated a focus on "uplifting stories of business, industry, and commerce" and biographies of American heroes, sports figures, and political leaders in place of stories of gangsters and kept women.

This endorsement of "realistic" subject matter highlights the competing conceptions of realism that would become central to the argument for formally separating entertainment from educational films. On one hand, entertainment pictures that are based on real people or events are considered to be morally uplifting; on the other hand, educational pictures that actually depict real events as they occur (in other words, films that document an unmediated profilmic reality) are considered to be morally corrosive, despite the fact that these real images might form the basis for an acceptable historical dramatization. Thus, the contradiction (or hypocrisy) of the code be-comes apparent, as the only forms of entertainment that it deems acceptable "influences in the life of a nation"[28] are those with little relation to reality.

By the beginning of 1933, over forty national organizations had passed resolutions condemning the film industry and demanding federal control and elimination of block booking.[29] The opposition to "immorality" in the movies, which had been articulated by state and municipal censorship boards and by various social pressure groups through the mid-1920s, had only led to the creation of nominal self-regulation measures by the film in-dustry. The demands for federal censorship did result in three series of con-gressional hearings—in 1914, 1916, and 1926—but all were unsuccessful from the reform perspective.[30] The "Thirteen Points" of 1921, the "Formula" of 1924, the "open door" policy of the Hays Office Department of Public Re-lations in 1925, the eleven "Don'ts" and twenty-five "Be Carefuls" in 1927, and the first Production Code in 1930 were all meant to serve as evidence that the studios earnestly shared the moral outrage expressed by so many reform-minded citizens.[31] However, the lack of enforcement mechanisms soon made apparent the superficiality of these measures, and, as a result, the film industry's apologetic stance toward protest groups appeared increas-ingly disingenuous. By the time the Payne Fund Studies were published in 1933, the discourse of reform had reached fever pitch, and the morally minded American public was prepared to embrace the scientifically legiti-mated crusade against morally infectious motion pictures.[32]

THE PAYNE FUND STUDIES: EDUCATION VERSUS ENTERTAINMENT

The widely publicized debates of the early 1930s over the effects of motion pictures on their viewers were of obvious economic interest to the Hollywood studios, whose very livelihood was under assault. But they also had impor-tant consequences for producers of educational films—particularly health education films—as the content and the mode of address of motion pic-tures were under investigation and the subject matter of health films was becoming increasingly controversial. In this period, the first rigorous social scientific studies of motion pictures were undertaken, in an attempt to pro-vide empirical evidence of the physiological and psychological impact of film viewing on youth. A central node of inquiry was the spectator's ability to distinguish "reality" from "fiction" in the movie-viewing experience.

Various conceptions of the psychological effects of movie viewing were already in circulation long before the topic became the subject of scientific inquiry. For instance, the federal government's involvement in film production during World Wars One and Two was motivated by the assumption that motion picture viewing constituted an ideal scenario for both logistical and ideological instruction. But while the government viewed the spectators' suggestibility as essential to their training, the film reform movement viewed this vulnerability as cause for alarm. The occasion of spectatorship was regarded as an opportunity for moral contagion, and implicit in the reformers' assumption that motion pictures have identifiable "effects" on their viewers was a theory not only of the relationship between film and conduct but also of the relationship between film and history. Rather than passively reflecting a historical period, films were thought actively to shape the course of history by controlling the behavior of moviegoers, in a model of spectatorship that imagined the Hollywood moguls conspiring to control the audience by "injecting" them with a potent dose of propaganda as they sat in the dark.[33] In the 1930s, the Payne Fund Studies popularized a crucial and enduring articulation of the injection theory of film spectatorship.

The debates over whether motion pictures are transmitters of education or purveyors of entertainment are as old as the history of film regulation and censorship, which is, in turn, as old as the medium itself. However, in the early 1930s, the debates acquired a newfound prestige and a greatly expanded audience when the Motion Picture Research Council commissioned the Payne Fund Studies. The studies consist of thirteen scientific investigations, twelve of which were published between 1933 and 1935, along with the summary of the findings, Henry James Forman's *Our Movie Made Children*, which was published for popular consumption in 1933.[34] The studies examine the effects of movies on conduct from a variety of perspectives, questioning the significance of variables such as age, race, ethnicity, gender, religion, and socioeconomic class in determining a viewer's response to different genres and to specific images, stereotypes, and episodes within particular films.[35] These investigations were promoted as the first serious attempts to measure systematically and scientifically the psychological effects of movies on viewers, with the hope of ascertaining the most effective method of censoring motion pictures that contained potentially harmful material.[36]

Despite the claims of the studies' objectivity, *Our Movie Made Children* accuses motion pictures of corrupting the nation's youth, and when the book became a national best seller, it provided film reformers with seemingly irrefutable evidence that the content of the movies was damaging and needed to be sharply restricted.[37] While the Payne Fund Studies formed the center of this debate, two other texts were also of particular importance: Milton Anderson's *The Modern Goliath* and a collection of essays titled *The Movies on Trial*.[38] With the publication of this group of texts, the proverbial floodgates were opened; debates about "movies and morals" filled the popular press. An enormous number of film treatises was published between 1933 and World War Two, and with the expanded use of motion pictures for the training of troops during the war, the "science" of audiovisual education accounted for an equally voluminous output of treatises after the war.[39]

But the central terms of the debate were clearly defined by the Payne Fund Studies.[40] This set of sociological investigations argued that motion pictures have a civic obligation to morally elevate reality and, thus, to morally elevate their viewers. The authors of the studies concluded that in their present state, the movies do not fulfill this function but rather debase reality, dragging the audience down with them. The Payne Fund Studies argued that motion pictures provide both entertainment and education for their audiences, but on the whole the content of the movies is largely "unwholesome," and therefore the movies provide an education in "immorality" for their viewers.

As a result of their investigations of the boundaries between fantasy and reality, the social scientists determined not only that the majority of motion pictures redefined "realism" along dangerous lines by naturalizing immoral, criminal activities but also that viewers tended to imitate the version of "reality" that they saw onscreen. The popularized summary of the studies cautions, "Many educators and laymen alike . . . have had a conviction that the motion picture with its immense range and vast reach falls little short of being a supplementary educational system of our nation. Indeed, some laymen have gone so far as to believe that the motion picture vies in importance with the national school system."[41] Thus, the studies claim that it is the educational function of film that must be scrutinized, since "unwholesome" entertainments are only damaging to the extent that they are imitated by the audience.

The debates of the 1930s emphasize the linkage of realism with film's educational value, regardless of whether the education is in criminal techniques or brotherly love. In the industry's and reformers' efforts to purify the realm of entertainment pictures, two diametrically opposed and morally saturated versions of realism are articulated: a negative form of realism is associated with the immorality of excessively graphic content (such as representations of childbirth or war), while a positive form of realism is linked with the morality of artistically elevated fiction (as in wholesome studio pictures such as *Beau Geste*, a film that is now widely seen as sadistic and homoerotic, but which nonetheless received accolades from the Catholic Legion of Decency).[42] Within this logic, the educational potential of film must be negated in order for the studios to produce films that fulfill the positive, uplifting potential of the medium. Thus, while the discourse of motion picture reform elevates education over entertainment, the institutional implementation of the reformers' demands actually devalues education, aligning it with films that should be excluded from mainstream exhibition venues. Even more ironically, the most celebrated studio pictures are those that deal with purportedly real subjects such as historical dramatizations, while the most reviled are those that depict the actual traumatic events that invest such fictionalized dramatizations with their narrative drive.

Our Movie-Made Children opens with and frequently repeats three key facts meant to alarm the American public: at least 77 million Americans go to the movies each week; 28 million viewers are children and adolescents; and the prevailing motion picture themes that this audience absorbs deal with love, sex, and crime.[43] Given these statistics, Forman argues that if this many Americans, and especially young Americans, are seeing this many movies, then surely these viewers must be affected by the movies they see. Furthermore, if most of the movies treat lurid subject matter, then the motion pictures must have a negative effect on their viewers, and because the audience is so large, the movies must also have a negative effect on the entire American culture. The implications of this rationale are that the motion pictures function as an unregulated educational system and that the national scope of the motion picture "problem," with its detrimental effects on our nation's physiology and psychology, qualifies as a public health menace and must be combated as such. Within *Our Movie Made Children* and in the broader discourse of reform, the recurring metaphors for the effects of movie viewing collapse three major institutions of the public sphere: the motion pictures, the educational system, and the public health service, unifying all three in a discourse of social control that becomes, in the postwar period, the discourse of world health.[44]

The popular and social scientific treatises of the 1930s constructed motion pictures as a problem of public hygiene in three key ways: the dark, dirty, unventilated, smoky, and crowded theaters come under assault as contaminated environments in which contagion could spread; the loosening of morals associated with film spectatorship links their detrimental influence with that of urban vices such as alcohol consumption; and finally, the popular descriptions of the impact of movie viewing aligns perception with bodily ingestion, linking the consumption of motion pictures with the consumption of milk, meat, and other federally regulated food products. Ironically, film is the privileged medium of education for institutions of public health, but it is also identified as a source of the very contaminations that public health organizations were designed to combat. This view of motion picture theaters as polluted environments where invisible contagions spread was explicitly recognized by the Payne Fund researchers in a proposed (but never completed) study entitled "Special Case Studies of Motion Picture Theaters which are known or suspected to be Foci of Moral Infection."[45]

In keeping with the notion that movies materially shape the physiognomy of their viewers, Forman conceives of the motion picture as a tool that writes upon or sculpts the viewer's subjectivity: "If . . . they had received whatever they had gleaned from the screen with the pliability of wax, they were found to be retaining it, as the phrase goes, with the durability of marble."[46] It is the material quality of this psychological impact that invests the motion pictures with their reality effect and renders vulnerable viewers (not surprisingly, women, immigrants, and children) incapable of distinguishing fantasy from reality. Ironically (or perhaps, disingenuously), even Will Hays, as head of the Motion Picture Producers and Distributors of America (MPPDA), adopted the attitude that children's minds are highly vulnerable to molding by the intense stimulus of the motion pictures. In a suitably melodramatic tone, Hays warned that "this industry must have toward that sacred thing, the mind of a child, toward that clean and virgin thing, the unmarked slate, the same responsibility, the same care about the impressions made upon it that the best clergyman or the most inspired teacher of youth would have."[47]

The spectator's inability to distinguish truth from fiction is attributed to the cinema's unique potency as an educational tool, and this potency derives from the conception of film spectatorship as a process of contagion. As the innocent viewer sits captivated by the excessively real images onscreen, the invisible germs of immorality and social disease penetrate the child's bodily boundaries through the distinctively permeable membrane of vision. Film spectatorship materially impacts the body of the viewer and thus qualifies as a problem of public health: "The seeing of a motion picture is for young children a powerful emotional experience that affects their young brains and nerves with almost the force of an electric charge. . . . That virtually none remains unaffected and all are powerfully affected by what they see on the screen, is a fact not only of scientific importance, but of the highest hygienic significance."[48] While the movies are frequently described as educational tools, they are attributed an intensity far surpassing that of the average textbook—an intensity that often leads to one of Forman's favored concepts from the studies: "emotional possession." As defined in *Movies, Delinquency, and Crime,*

> Certain types of motion pictures may indirectly influence delinquent and criminal behavior by inducing emotional possession. . . . the inciting of impulses, the arousing of a given emotion, a relaxing of ordinary control, and so an increased readiness to yield to the impulses aroused. These states of mind and feeling come, usually, as a result of the individual "losing himself" in the picture, or becoming deeply preoccupied with its drama or movement.[49]

In this scenario, the spectator is unconsciously infected by the emotions displayed onscreen and later exhibits the symptoms of contagion by reenacting the contaminating scenes. The Payne Fund researchers feared that repeated outbreaks of this form of excitement could develop into a permanent and detrimental behavior pattern (akin to a chronic infectious disease), in which the individual would consistently view herself or himself in the role of the gold digger or gangster, acting in accord with that character type. This loss of distance between subject and object, self and other was seen as an indirect way in which the movies were a cause of immorality and crime. For the Payne Fund Studies, it is the physiological manifestation of emotion, the possibility of losing control of one's body that imbues the movie viewing experience with such intense and therefore dangerous consequences.

Because the mental impact of the movies was understood as leading directly to the performance of that which has been imprinted on the mind, "education" was implicitly defined by the Payne Fund Studies as the compulsion to imitate that which has been visually ingested. Thus, the movies were described as a "school of conduct" that was competing with the traditional educational system for the audience's attention, as in the following quote: "For the visual aid, the semblance of living actuality presented on the screen, is almost incalculably powerful. . . . Obviously, in these conditions, the film must emerge as one of the most potent of all educational instruments."[50] According to the Payne Fund Studies, the imitative aspect of this educational system derives from its realism, its ability to represent fantastical events and characters as "true to life," and it is this very realism that authorizes the regulation of motion pictures in the national interest.

The conception of the cinema as a threat to national values and the "American way of life" is demonstrated by the rhetorical linkage of the unregulated chaos of motion pictures with a premodern, uncivilized society: "The screen becomes one of the most powerful single instruments in the education of our population. Yet an African tribe could scarcely have used it more irresponsibly."[51] This linkage of uncontrolled motion picture content with implicitly uncontrolled—because racialized—behavior is subtly suggestive of the reform movement's desire to regulate the behavior of the non-white immigrants whose bodies filled the urban motion picture theaters of the United States.[52] As noted earlier in this chapter, the mass immigration to the United States from 1880 to 1924 was widely perceived as an onslaught of diseased bodies threatening to penetrate the borders of an otherwise pure nation, and consequently the racial and national difference of the immigrant body was regarded as a vector of contagion that must be contained through public health measures. The linkage of the "African tribe" with the motion picture problem thus points to another key metaphor in the debates over education versus entertainment: cinema as immigrant, "alien" public health menace.

The treatment of motion pictures themselves as vectors of contagion was recognized in *Our Movie Made Children*, but prior to the publication of the Payne Fund Studies summary, Reverend Short, Director of the Motion Picture Research Council (the funding agency for the studies), warned Forman against articulating an explicitly antimovie perspective. However, the collected papers of the Motion Picture Research Council reveal not only that Short shared Forman's negative attitude toward the film industry, but also that he clearly conceived of the "movie problem" in terms of the discourse of contagion.[53] One of Short's letters demonstrates the "venereal theory of film influence": "An evil girl in a community will infect a whole group of boys in spite of the fact that there are good girls in the same community."[54] Similarly, an "evil" movie will infect an otherwise "good" audience, turning them into a group of delinquents: "For [bad girls] the movies constitute an education along the left-hand or primrose path of life, to the wreckage of their own lives and to the detriment and cost of society. . . . The road to delinquency, in a few words, is heavily dotted with movie addicts, and obviously, it needs no crusaders or preachers or reformers to come to this conclusion."[55]

According to Forman, the end result of moviegoing is "moral turpitude," and therefore motion picture attendance is a vice from which good citizens must abstain, as they would abstain from any other addictive substance. The effects of movie viewing are linked not only to moral degeneracy, but also to physiological impairment, as in a study of the effects of movie viewing on sleep:

> If a child shows decreased motility after a movie or sleep loss, this greater quiet may be a quiet of the same type *produced by soporific drugs*, not a more restful, recuperative sleep. . . . The significant increases of fatigue, whether induced by sleep impairment following the movies, from overwork, from narcotic drugs or alcohol, or any source of oxygen deprivation, are detrimental to health and growth, not only because of their known physiological consequences, but also because of the fact that the

important inhibitions which serve to prevent misconduct are weakened. Frequent indulgence may lead to the formation of the habit of craving further indulgence. The best hygienic regulations for children should therefore include, among other things, only infrequent attendance at selected types of motion picture programmes.[56]

The conception of motion pictures as materially impacting a viewer's mind leads to the metaphoric slippage between film consumption and ingestion of other substances into the body, as we have seen with the comparison of movies and alcohol. This slippage is significant not only because it aligns motion pictures with invisible contagions, but also because of the sexual implications of this type of bodily boundary crossing. In the popular summary of the Payne Fund Studies, the invisible effects of the movies within the body of the viewer are linked to the demand for federal regulation of consumption in the public sphere: "Much has been done by way of safeguarding the purity and integrity of water supplies, of food and drugs. The motion picture presents itself as nothing less than a food universally but confusedly ingested by the human mind."[57] The physiological effects of motion picture attendance are thus conceived as a source of both sustenance and contamination, an almost literal "injection" of moral contagion. Thus, Forman's explanation of why "young criminals and delinquents" are more vulnerable to the negative effects of "bad" movies than to the positive effects of "good" movies emphasizes the inoculation factor: "Their environment . . . as well as their long continued and promiscuous movie-going with no selection other than their own tastes and proclivities has virtually immunized them to the good and sensitized them to the others."[58] Ironically, the movies were seen as both cause and cure for contagion, and the films that were produced for the specific purpose of preventing the spread of disease were considered just as harmful as the films that seemed to provoke the contaminating behavior in the first place.

"A SUBJECT MOST OBJECTIONABLE FOR PRESENTATION IN ENTERTAINMENT MOTION PICTURE THEATERS"

The popularized summary of the Payne Fund Studies presented an overall view of the motion pictures as a problem to be solved by regulating the content of the movies and the demographic makeup of the audience. The Catholic Legion of Decency, a religious reform group, was mobilized specifically to support these aims and combat the "motion picture problem" by distributing ratings of the morality of current movies in churches and organizing boycotts of offensive pictures playing at local theaters. Since the fundamental assumption underlying the legion's campaign was that certain kinds of pictures have an adverse moral effect on at least some of the people who view them, the legion's tactics were based on an estimation of the mental and moral caliber of the audience. Their primary considerations were the age composition of the audience and the heterogeneous social environment of the movie theater; the latter concern directly impinged on the domain of health films.[59] In the reformers' view, the educational film was linked to films that dealt with venereal disease, drug and alcohol addiction, and the "white slave trade," most of which were condemned because "the Legion maintains that an audience whose social character is partially determined by the fact that both sexes are gathered together to be entertained is not properly receptive to instruction in sex hygiene."[60] The legion maintained this position regardless of the quality of the picture, though it did make a separate classification for documentary films dealing with childbirth, with the reservation that "the film is not suited to general exhibition in the theater." These concerns reflect the Payne Fund Studies' preoccupation with the possibility that sex or romance movies would induce an outbreak of immoral viewer responses (sexual or emotional possession) in the theater itself.

The legion continued to rate films well after its initial campaign for institutionalized censorship succeeded in reinforcing the Production Code in 1934, and its condemnation of the "sex education" exploitation blockbuster *Mom and Dad* (1944) typifies the organization's approach to the material context of exhibition and the problematic heterogeneity of the audience. In the legion's view, "This film deals with a subject most objectionable for presentation in entertainment motion picture theaters. Moreover, the treatment of the subject as presented in the film is most objectionable for entertainment motion picture audiences. It ignores completely essential and supernatural values associated with questions of this nature."[61] This review is typical in its condemnation of explicit cinematic discussion of sexual matters and "social diseases." The legion's critique is based on two principles: first, the topics demand a spiritual treatment, not a medical or social one. The legion was concerned that secular films and doctors would usurp religious authority to define proper sexuality—for the Catholic Legion of Decency, sex is a religious issue because it is a moral issue. Second, the reviewers assume, as did the Payne Fund researchers, that most members of motion picture audiences ingest the images projected on the screen with no comprehension of the context from which they are derived. Thus, in viewing a documentary on syphilis, a viewer would only be influenced by the fact that the movie was about sex, not by the discussion of the devastating venereal disease that resulted. These reservations about the various constituencies of the "social environment" derive from concerns about the mixing of sexes, classes, ethnic groups, and age groups in the motion picture theaters, and the Legion of Decency concluded—and convinced the Production Code Administration to agree—that such unorthodox mixing would inevitably lead to immorality.

The sexualized collapse of motion pictures, (immoral) education, and public health reveals the centrality of fears about bodily border crossing and contagion to the models of film spectatorship that ultimately led to the revision of the Production Code in 1934. With the standardization of film censorship codes in the MPPDA's various self-regulation measures, "sex hygiene," "venereal diseases," "surgical operations," "scenes of actual childbirth, in fact or in silhouette," and other "sex perversions" were deemed "not proper subjects for theatrical motion pictures."[62] As Martin Pernick has demonstrated, the Production Code not only established the boundaries of cinematic propriety through institutionalized censorship, it also formalized the distinctions between what is now known as the classical Hollywood film and other genres of audiovisual representation. In his discussion of early cinematic representations of euthanasia, Pernick argues that

> medical films such as *The Black Stork* spurred the construction of distinctions between "entertainment" and such genres as education, propaganda, and exploitation films, and led to the physical segregation of the places where these genres could be shown. . . ."Nontheatrical," the catchall term for any film whose aspirations went beyond pleasant entertainment, indicates the extent to which genre and geography coincided to keep alternatives to Hollywood in their place.[63]

The expanded Production Code of 1934 contained a new requirement that films with plotlines that depended on crime or sin must contain "compensating moral value" to justify the representation of immoral activities. As Gregory Black has explained, "This meant that these films must have a good character who spoke as a voice for morality, a character who clearly told the criminals or sinner that he or she was wrong. Each film must contain a stern moral lesson: regeneration, suffering, and punishment."[64] The code was intended unilaterally to purify the movies, regardless of the specific "immorality" they might contain—thus the obscure requirement that nothing "subversive of the fundamental law of the land" could be depicted onscreen. Instead, Hollywood movies would promote "social spirit" and "patriotism" and "not confuse audiences with a 'cynical contempt for conventions' nor too vivid a recreation of the 'realism of problems' encountered in life."[65]

In addition to explicitly forbidding activities deemed excessively realistic and thus morally inappropriate, the Production Code also aimed to address other public relations problems that had developed with the advent of talking pictures in the late 1920s. To film censors and reformers, synchronized sound raised cinema's potential realism in dangerous ways; explicit dialogue about contemporary social themes, including the affairs of gangsters and "loose" women, was perceived as a threatening source of instruction in criminal immorality. As Ruth Vasey has shown, the MPPDA attempted to mitigate cinema's increasing potential for offense by deliberately introducing ambiguity into films, "to allow multiple interpretations by multiple audiences," and thus ensure a continued widespread (and innocent) reception of Hollywood films at home and abroad.[66] One effect of this intentional ambiguity was a revision of Hollywood's treatment of physical and cultural difference:

> "Foreignness" became less clearly associated with particular ethnic and national groups and became abstracted into an amorphous category of the alien, so that specific interest groups could find fewer grounds for complaint. Even geography became less distinct, with "mythical kingdoms" often standing in for exotic locations in Latin America, Africa, Europe, and the Far East, so that film commerce abroad would not be affected by the casual insult of national stereotyping.[67]

Thus, the Production Code eliminated graphic representations of the body and explicit commentary on configurations of geopolitical power from entertainment films, relegating such "realistic" subject matter to nonentertainment film forms. Hollywood could no longer directly address medical issues, nor could it specifically represent a view (however distorted) of international relations—both forms of audiovisual representation were consigned to the "nontheatrical" realm.

Within the broad rubric of nontheatrical films, further divisions exist that emphasize the concepts of realism and actuality in order to differentiate between documentary and other kinds of films. As Philip Rosen has argued, the term "documentary" acquired a specific cinematic definition largely through the writings of filmmaker John Grierson, who is credited with the initial use of the term in reference to film form in his "First Principles of Documentary" (1932–34), published contemporaneously with the Payne Fund Studies. In this piece, Grierson sets about defining documentary as an elevated art form, not to be confused with the use of film simply to capture reality. As Rosen argues:

> [Grierson's] preferred category of filmmaking excludes such "films made from natural materials" as travelogues, newsreels, "magazine items," and other short "interests" or "lecture films," as well as scientific and educational films. Beyond such nonfiction film types, "one begins to wander into the world of documentary proper, into the only world in which documentary can hope to achieve the ordinary virtues of an art. Here, we pass from the plain (or fancy) descriptions of natural material, to arrangements, rearrangements, and creative shapings of it."[68]

The practice of cinematic documentary is thus self-consciously defined as an aestheticization of reality, an addition to the unvarnished capturing of images and sounds that characterizes such allegedly debased forms of "nonfiction" cinematic representation as newsreels and public health films. The movement to regulate motion picture content had consistently targeted crime and romance pictures as well as medical and health films that were subjected to codes of "aesthetic censorship." As a result, motion picture exhibition was separated into artful entertainment genres on one hand and debased instructional films on the other.

A significant component of the motion picture reform discourse was the distinction, in definitions of the boundaries of decency, between what constitutes decency for an audience of the general public and what constitutes decency for a restricted audience. Film censors and film aestheticians were both invested, though for different reasons, in distinguishing art from "reality," and in the process, both groups identified instructional and educational films as their negative examples—as the types of films that produce an undesirably unvarnished form of realism. On one hand, then, the regulators of Hollywood exhibition practices demanded a separation of entertainment from excessively realistic, aesthetically unpleasing "nonfiction" programs such as public health films. On the other hand, practitioners of the "nonfiction" form of documentary elevated their own work above the (again, aesthetically unpleasing) form of "actualities" such as public health films. In both cases, entertainment and documentary are aligned with aesthetic pleasure and opposed to realism, the burden of the artistically impoverished educational film. And yet, different versions of "realism" have been crucially important to both classical Hollywood film and the history of documentary film.

Significantly, Rosen notes that according to the *Oxford English Dictionary*, the cultural use of the term "documentary" had expanded to include noncinematic meanings by the late 1950s, which suggests "a cultural conjuncture *requiring* some designation of the field [Grierson] named: an arena of meaning centering on the authority of the real founded in the indexical trace, various forms of which were rapidly disseminated at all levels of industrial and now postindustrial culture."[69] This cultural "requirement" is answered not only by the widespread use (and official recognition) of the term "documentary" by the postwar period, but also by the fascination with the indexical in audiovisual representations of a contemporaneous cultural conjuncture, namely, the epistemology of world health. As a mode of representation aligned with "realism" and distinguished from "entertainment" and "documentary," public health films acquired (almost by default) a privileged relation to indexicality. And yet, this relation was far from unproblematic; while the genre did accept its designation as the repository of realism, it also struggled anxiously to produce indexical representations of a subject that eludes such capture—that is, the spread of contagious disease. It is precisely the location of public health films within this "sociocultural matrix bestowing authority on purported conveyances of a real,"[70] that lends relevance to the films as part of a broader discursive formation, and their historical importance is only enhanced by their position as the privileged media of self-promotion within international health surveillance organizations.

After 1934, health film themes were explicitly censored from entertainment pictures by the revised Production Code and were therefore no longer considered appropriate material for exhibition to a general, mixed audience in a public theater. This meant that educational films would have to develop different distribution mechanisms and find new locations for screenings. The effects of these changes became especially evident after World War Two, when audiovisual technologies became extraordinarily popular as teaching tools within public schools. But even before then, the reinforcement of the boundaries of decency through institutionalized regulation of commercial representation was seen as vital to preventing moral contagion in the public sphere.

By separating education from entertainment in the process of institutionalizing the Production Code, the social reformers of the 1930s, the Legion of Decency, and the MPPDA subjected entertainment pictures to intense scrutiny and heavily enforced moralizing, leaving educational films (comparatively) free of such restrictions. Because educational films were not subject to the "compensating moral value" requirement, they were able to represent sexual and other "improper" topics unambiguously and without being hampered by a fictionalized narrative rationalization. And yet, the removal of such restrictions from the educational film did not result in a radical development of the genre, free from the constraints of the classical Hollywood form and style. On the contrary, public health and Hollywood films of the postwar period were each increasingly influenced by the conventions of the other mode of representation, as the comparison of *Panic in the Streets* and *Prevention of the Introduction of Diseases from Abroad* attests. And in the case of public health films, the freedom from one set of institutional regulations only led to subjection to another institutional ideology—the discourse of world health.

The end result of this logic is the polarization of education and entertainment in debates over regulation of the film industry, with the consequent elimination of the "educational" function from "entertainment" films, enforced through the literal separation of commercial entertainment venues and noncommercial educational exhibition sites. But the attempted separation of public health and Hollywood modes of representation is ultimately circumvented through the different genres' shared participation in broader discourses of visuality and disease. Thus, the official articulation of boundaries between these spheres of discourse did not produce rigid demarcations between health science and mass culture but, rather, resulted in the intensified permeation of each sphere with the other's modes of representation. That is, rather than clearly defining the boundaries between public health and Hollywood films, the separation of their production, distribution, exhibition, and regulation ultimately resulted in the interweaving of discourses of world health and popular representational forms. Despite the rejection of the educational film by purveyors of mass entertainment *and* by practitioners of the documentary arts, the dominant representational forms of the public health film (and the ideals underlying those forms) permeated popular culture in the postwar period and continue to do so today.

CHAPTER 2

"Noninfected but Infectible":

CONTAGION AND THE BOUNDARIES OF THE VISIBLE

Epidemics break out, far from the known infected areas. Country to country, continent to continent, the deadly cargo of microbes is transported, menacing on a vast scale the very existence of humanity.

The Eternal Fight (1948)

WORLD HEALTH AND THE DIALECTICS OF VISIBILITY

AND INVISIBILITY

Even a cursory glance at contemporary U.S. film and television reveals a cultural obsession with contagious disease, both as a biological threat and as a rhetorical trope describing the spread of any number of insidious, malevolent forces across the globe. Nightly newscasts perpetually reiterate the central problem: strategic and technological failure in the face of an invisible enemy. While this danger is often construed as a novel feature of the emerging geopolitical reality known as globalization, the current interest is only the latest articulation of a long-standing and continually evolving epistemological formation that has come to dominate key areas of cultural production in the United States since World War Two. At the conceptual core of this formation is a preoccupation with the boundaries of visibility—a concern that links the invisibility of contagion to other potentially invisible aspects of identity, particularly race and sexuality, in an effort to pin the elusive contaminant to a concrete embodiment of "otherness."

With its aim of visually representing the transnational spread of contagious disease, the postwar project of global health surveillance is heavily invested in monitoring physical and national boundaries. As a result, the films produced by international health organizations compulsively pose (and attempt to solve) the problem of visualizing invisible contagions. Within this archive of films, the human body is a recurring object of anxious attention—

it is the site where the global flow of information and commodities is joined to the global flow of contagious diseases. Through this juncture, the movement of bodies and commerce across geopolitical boundaries is conflated with the infectious transgression of bodily boundaries. The threat posed by international exchange thus resides in the potentially undetected passage of invisible contaminants across institutionally regulated borders, as globalization becomes both vector and antidote for contagious disease.[1] This chapter will examine the use of motion pictures by international health surveillance organizations (such as the u.s. Public Health Service and the World Health Organization) as technologies of instruction, education, and discursive production. As I will demonstrate in my discussion of two postwar public health films—*Hemolytic Streptococcus Control* (a 1945 United States Navy training film) and *The Eternal Fight* (a 1948 United Nations film)—a dialectic of visibility and invisibility pervades the films that attempt to represent contagious disease. In these films, the tension between indexical representation of the body and the impossibility of visualizing potential threats to that body's integrity reveals the paranoia about maintaining organic national boundaries that underlies the supposed confidence of the globally hegemonic postwar United States. Moreover, the repeated representation of bodily dissolution in these films highlights their connection to contemporaneous popular cinematic forms engaged in the anxious production of coherent spectatorial subjects.[2]

The problem of invisible mobility is consistently posed in audiovisual representations of contagion through two distinct and opposing modes of visual realism. I will call these poles "indexical" and "artificial," though as we will see, both poles strive for indexicality, and both have a fundamentally artificial relationship to "the real."[3] The indexical pole can only secure its realism through an ideological (that is, discursive, not mechanical) relation to the profilmic, while the artificial pole asserts its realism through extrafilmic means of revealing the hidden truth of the profilmic. More specifically, the indexical mode of representation employs visible stigma of bodily otherness—that is, "obvious" signs of racial and sexual difference—as signs of contagion, while the artificial mode of representation utilizes the techniques of voiceover and animation to trace the paths of contagion between individuals, nations, and continents. Thus, the films under investigation here construct meaning through their oscillation between two poles; the first invokes race and sexuality as signifiers of a "real" whose self-evident truth functions indexically, as an unmediated document of essential difference.[4] This mode of representation establishes its own authenticity and realism by treating race and sexuality as irreducible, foundational categories of identity (or otherness) that can be captured simply by pointing a camera and shooting.[5] In other words, this pole attributes to the surface of the body—and consequently, to the surface of the *image* of that body—a transparency which creates the impression of unfettered access to an interior corporeal truth.

Within the audiovisual discourse of world health, the racial and sexual features of these transparently legible bodies perform the crucial function of linking bodily otherness with implied contaminations that are nationally specific in origin. In the postwar period, racial difference is collapsed with national difference, and the threat of physical and geopolitical penetration by invisible contagions is conceived as a sexualized attack. The films that utilize marked bodies as vectors of contagion emphatically draw attention to the infectious difference between the diseased bodies and their imperial others (often distinguished by their whiteness, masculinity, and wealth). The body captured on film is essentially coextensive with the profilmic body; image and object are indistinguishable in their materiality. Thus, these films partake of a Bazinian conceptualization of realism, in which "the photographic image is the object itself, the object freed from the conditions of time and space that govern it."[6] While this passage refers most directly to the indexical quality of mechanical reproduction through photography, it also implicitly claims that within photographic representation, the relationship between signifier and signified is fundamentally unambiguous. It is precisely through their reliance on this form of indexical realism that the public health films that conflate bodily difference with disease assert their own objectivity. By maintaining that racial and sexual difference transparently correlate to contagion, these films establish their own ideological structures of signification as universal truths and, thus, as authentic documents of realism.

At the other, "artificial" representational pole is the attempt to constitute realism through nonindexical means; here, animation and voiceover function as cinematic manipulations that affirm their authenticity by foregrounding their artifice. In this mode of representation, the techniques that have been celebrated since the invention of cinema as the medium's unique attributes—its ability to expand and contract space and time, and its power to visually represent that which is invisible to the naked eye—are pushed to the extreme. In contrast to the early medical films that showcased microscopy, the later public health films under investigation here push image-sound relations beyond the point of severance, replacing enlargements with animated sequences, and the separation of the audio from the visual is promoted as the means by which truth can be secured. As Tom Gunning has argued, the films produced prior to the consolidation of the classical Hollywood style partook of an "aesthetic of astonishment," in which pleasure revolved around the fascination of seeing previously unimaginable views, including enlargements of bacteria and other revelations of the invisible, disease-carrying microbes that surround us.[7] But the institutionalization of "aesthetic censorship" in the Production Codes of the 1930s separated earlier health films, with their scientific aesthetic of astonishment, from the films under examination here, which disallow such fascination with unembellished actuality by turning to animation for their revelatory moments of truth.[8] Thus, while the pole that naturalizes race and sexuality guarantees veracity (or realism) through its *lack* of mediation, this second pole guarantees its documentary truth precisely through its refusal to utilize *any* preexisting profilmic reality, turning instead to nonindexical means of creating images and sounds.[9] These attempts to produce spectatorial inoculation through representations of contagion are surprisingly dependent upon the visual and aural dissection of the very human body whose desired unity drives the organization of images and sounds in classical Hollywood-style realism. And yet, instead of producing incompatible versions of embodied realism, the institutional and ideological intersections of public health and cinema create a broader discursive field that absorbs and simultaneously promotes these contradictory visions of the public bodies that will accomplish (or undermine) the ideals of world health.

REPRODUCING REALISM: BACTERIOLOGY AND THE INVENTION OF CINEMA

The history of audiovisual production by global health surveillance organizations is linked to both the history of medicine and the history of early cinema; indeed, recent scholarship has located the interconnections between these fields within a broader surveillant impulse in late-nineteenth- and early-twentieth-century modernity.[10] But while such work has begun to account for the ideologies produced through medicine and cinema, the substantial intensification of this institutional intersection in the postwar period has not received sufficient attention. As two institutions that fundamentally transformed (and were transformed by) the public sphere in the early twentieth century, motion pictures and medicine—particularly the public health branch of medicine—constitute an important intersection of discourses about regulation of the individual and the national body, especially in the period of mass immigration from 1880 to 1924. As the prehistory to the postwar practice of world health will show, there are not only important linkages between the history of public health and the history of cinema, but these parallel histories have together formed a self-contradictory though nonetheless culturally dominant discourse on the mutually constitutive processes of modernization and sanitation of the public sphere. In its reliance upon moving images to visually represent invisible paths of contagion, this discourse is informed by both public health and cinematic imaginations of the presence of disease in the processes of exchange that characterize the consumer culture of modernity.

To contextualize the intersection of the surveillant gaze and the cinematic discourse of contagion, this chapter will examine some key moments of institutional and representational intersection in the histories of public health and cinema: the "bacteriological revolution" of the 1880s, the invention of cinema in the 1890s, the Spanish American War in 1898, and World Wars One and Two. With the increasingly elaborate mobilization of bodies across geopolitical borders from the late nineteenth century through the mid-twentieth, the technologies of monitoring and visually representing contagious disease became increasingly systematic in their modes of production. By tracing this history, I will demonstrate that the parallels between public health and cinematic institutionalization and representation emerge from historical concerns with invisible contagions that are linked to broader concerns about globalization. Moreover, the same anxiety that drives health surveillance organizations in their frustrated attempts to represent contagious disease is reproduced in the organizations' privileging of film as the medium whose unique ability to capture "the real" will enable the elusive invisible to be visualized. As I hope to demonstrate, film's supposedly privileged access to the real continually fails to secure an indexical image of contagion, and thus the audiovisual discourse of world health compulsively attempts and fails to visualize invisible disease. By explaining the historical roots of this compulsion, I will contextualize the contradictions that underlie the early intersections of public health and cinema—contradictions that are intensified in the proliferation of postwar audiovisual articulations of "world health."

The conceptual shift from miasma to bacteriology revolutionized medicine and public health in the 1880s. That is, the shift from the theory that miasma (a vaguely defined airborne substance implicitly linked to ethnic and economic degeneracy) caused disease to the theory that microscopic pathogenic organisms could be linked to specific illnesses transformed the fundamental conception of contagion in the late nineteenth century. The identification of the microscopic organisms that caused many widely feared (and lethal) diseases redefined the terrain of visibility and invisibility—a transformation that was further intensified by the invention of cinema in the following decade. However, the empirical evidence that the new representational technologies seemed to provide was no less ideological or irrational than the theory of miasma had been. As Alan Kraut has described this contradiction, "Even as many western Europeans and Americans were abandoning their belief in miasmas as the origin of disease and concentrating upon dirty, unhygienic conditions as the source of sickness, the foreign-born continued to be perceived as the most significant public health menace."[11] Despite the indexical qualities that were attributed to mechanical reproductions, the alliance of science and cinematography resulted in an expansion, not a reduction, of discursive production linking contagion to subjective interpretations of visible differences.

The identification of microorganisms finally enabled the concrete linkage of many deadly diseases to specific causes, which led, in turn, to the identification of specific disease carriers, specific modes of transmission, and, ultimately, to the development of vaccines and antitoxins.[12] This power to establish unambiguously the paths of contagion might have been the beginning of the end of the discursive linkage of disease and difference; scientific evidence could now prove that microbes without any national, ethnic, or class allegiances were the causes of disease, not their carriers. However, while these developments did enhance the social authority of medicine and consequently prompted the development of professional health departments in most urban centers, they did not break the historically entrenched linkage of disease and social difference. On the contrary, popular conceptions of racialized contagion structured the field of public health as it became increasingly standardized nationwide. While the development of microbiology enabled newly successful forms of treatment and prevention of contagious diseases based on laboratory identification of disease-causing microorganisms, techniques for quarantining the sick also became increasingly specialized. Thus, the practice of shoring up boundaries through quarantine that had characterized public health up to the 1880s was reasserted even at this seemingly revolutionary moment of discovery and expansion of knowledge. The breakthrough of microbiology certainly transformed the possibilities for preventing and curing diseases, but it did not dislodge the discourse of contagion that would continue to locate disease at the borders of the normative (white, literate, propertied, male) national body.[13]

With the development of microbiology in the 1880s and the invention of cinema in the 1890s, invisible contaminants gained materiality; through scientific classification and enlarged microscopic cinematography, the problem of visualizing contagion took on a distinct and increasingly popular representational form.[14] While the discourse of contagion would not reach its peak of popularity nor its most enduring iconography until World War Two (when it shifted from a national to a global discourse of world health), a new mode of imagining disease developed between the advent of bacteriology and the invention of cinema. In the late nineteenth century, cinema enabled medical imaging of bacteria in motion, and medical imaging, in turn, influenced the cinematic mode of representing disease.

Following close on the heels of the bacteriological revolution and the resultant professionalization of the fields of medicine and science, the Spanish American War in 1898 gave both the film industry and the field of public health their greatest impetus in moving toward large-scale, systematized production. For the motion picture industry, footage of (or even more importantly, reenactments of) scenes from the Spanish American War provided the materials for an enormous output of films, the popularity of which rescued the film industry from a likely fate as a short-lived novelty, becoming instead a massive industry.[15] Similarly, the quarantine inspection and disinfection of Spanish American War troops and their baggage required such an enormous mobilization of government public health administration that the event prompted the development of systematized and institutionalized armature against the threatened importation of yellow fever and other tropical diseases from Cuba, Puerto Rico, and other "exotic" locales.[16] The Spanish American War played a pivotal role in the development of public health and cinema, not only as a catalyst for the modernization of both industries, but also as an event that foregrounded the international spread of contagious disease as a problem of representation that would bind the fields of public health and cinema in their mutual regulation of the public sphere in the century to come.

As film historians have demonstrated, early motion picture audiences often described cinema as a magical curiosity, and one of the commonly cited attributes of this novelty was its ability to show things that the naked eye could not see, through manipulation of the film's speed (producing fast and slow motion) and through manipulation of the lens (producing enlargements and reductions of the image).[17] The ability to produce optical "tricks" through editing was another widely heralded feature of the new medium, as was stop-motion animation; both techniques were of crucial importance to the imagination of contagion, with its emphasis on visually representing the invisible. The fields of medicine and science made substantial use of these representational strategies; indeed, the very invention of cinema is attributed to scientists and inventors who were motivated by the desire for a camera that could capture movement in order to complete investigations of bodily motion in humans and animals.[18]

Further scientific value was ascribed to film's ability to represent microscopic organisms.[19] The early medical films that Tom Gunning associates with the "cinema of attractions" provided microscopic views of germs and thus offered a manipulated (through magnification) but nonetheless indexical image capturing a preexisting profilmic "truth" that would seem to provide an empirical foundation to the discourse of contagion.[20] Thus, a cinematic representation of microscopic bacteria could be inserted into a broader narrative of contagion, establishing a seemingly concrete linkage of images of a character's external appearance with images of the disease that lurks within. As Lisa Cartwright has shown, the scientific potential of cinema strongly influenced the medium's early uses: "The films of early-twentieth-century physiologists working in biology, zoology, neurology, and bacteriology constitute . . . evidence that, at the turn of the century, the motion picture apparatus was crucial in the emergence of a new set of optical techniques for social regulation. In laboratory culture, medical practice, and beyond, we see the emergence of a distinctly surveillant cinema."[21] And yet, these films also provide evidence of a founding (and ongoing) problem of public health: how to constitute the public sphere as an arena of bodily regulation, when the discipline's fundamental problem—the spread of contagious disease—is invisible to the naked eye.

While few health films from the 1890s and early 1900s survive today, records of early film production show an enormous output of popular films offering advice and instruction for all kinds of modern problems, including health issues. As Martin Pernick has demonstrated, "By 1915, only a decade after the first movie theaters had opened, the silent screen was filled with films on every aspect of medicine, from how to bathe the baby to how to avoid venereal disease; all part of an intense campaign to disseminate the discoveries of scientific public health and to promote the power and expertise of the scientific physician."[22] This trend continued until World War One, when commercial health films were supplemented by United States Public Health Service (USPHS) films produced for the military and the general public. In 1916, the federal government sponsored a nationwide "Safety First" campaign that traveled the country by rail. The program was mounted as an exhibit in nine thematically organized cars of a train, which visitors would enter at designated stops. The train included a Public Health Service car, whose exhibits were presented by a medical officer and two attendants, which displayed all of the current public health concerns—rat proofing, sanitary disposal of human waste, eradication of mosquitoes and flies—through motion pictures and lantern slides.[23]

The concerns of the USPHS also expanded to address specific issues arising out of World War One, such as malaria, the health of troops, the sanitation of camps and war industry areas, and venereal diseases. The historical simultaneity of World War One troop mobilization and the 1918–19 influenza pandemic consolidated the importance of the USPHS on a national and international scale. During this period, the institution organized the collection of health statistics, coordinated daily reports with state health departments, and mounted a nationwide public information campaign addressing influenza diagnosis, treatment, and prevention.[24] Through its institutional expansion, the USPHS established its domestic and global importance as an arbiter of geopolitical power by evaluating a population's relative "health" (in the United States and abroad) as an indicator of national development and modernization.[25]

After World War One ended in 1918, European immigration to the United States returned to the prewar highs, and this new flow of bodies was regulated even more closely than before the war.[26] Efforts to preserve the integrity of national borders through rigorous inspection of "alien" bodies were further institutionalized through legislation restricting foreign immigration to the United States. The 1924 Immigration Act establishing quotas for each nationality severely reduced the numbers of potentially contaminating bodies that could cross American borders, and to assist with this enhanced surveillance, in 1925 the USPHS began sending its own officers to directly examine prospective immigrants in their country of origin, at the time of their application for an American visa. This plan held until World War Two, when European immigration to the United States essentially ceased, but was reinstated at the end of the war.[27]

With millions of American soldiers crossing U.S. borders during the war, the exclusion of "alien" diseases became an even larger public concern than it had been when the problem was seen as only affecting immigrant carriers. Both foreign and American bodies had been linked with contamination upon traversing national boundaries since at least 1878, when the surgeon general began reporting statistics on venereal disease among merchant seamen. In an expansion of the xenophobia associated with "alien" exposures, the physical health of soldiers was subjected to intense scrutiny during World War One, and their sexual behavior became an important occasion for bodily surveillance. Exacerbating the concern over venereal diseases was the dramatic revelation of the overall poor health of the nation, as demonstrated by the results of draft examinations: of 2,510,706 potential draftees, 730,756 failed their fitness tests. A 1945 review in the *Journal of Health and*

Physical Education noted the effect of such figures on national morale: "The results of World War I draft examinations of young men 21 to 31 years of age shocked the nation. Almost all of the states enacted laws concerning health and physical education between 1918 and 1921."[28]

In fact, the prevention and treatment of venereal diseases spurred the first major film production by the u.s. government; the usphs was called upon to control the epidemic of sexually transmitted diseases among the troops, and the strategy deemed most effective and efficient was an educational program centering around a film, *Fit to Fight* (1918). The campaign was conducted in cooperation with state health departments, which distributed educational pamphlets to the film audiences.[29] Prior to the production of *Fit to Fight*, the armed services had been convinced of the persuasive powers of film by a commercial film production company, Bray Studios, who approached the War Department with the suggestion of using motion pictures for military training.[30] Although reportedly hesitant at first, upon viewing some animated slow-motion teaching films that Bray Studios had made as samples, the War Department commissioned a series of training films, sixty-two in all, that were in circulation until 1928.[31]

Significantly, a film produced by Bray Studios, *How Disease Is Spread*, contains one of the first cinematic representations of epidemiological mapping. This trope comes to play a crucial discursive role in the period after World War Two, but even in the early 1920s, the causal relationships between transportation, communication technologies, and the spread of disease were beginning to function as "common sense." One of the most significant developments of the interwar period — as evidenced by its centrality to the future iconography of world health — was the technological inauguration of the "Air Age." Charles Lindbergh became an international hero when he completed the first solo transatlantic air passage in 1927; the first international airport was constructed in the United States in 1928, linking Miami and Havana; and preceding both of these events, the Air Commerce Act of 1926 had empowered the usphs to "prevent the introduction of diseased persons and disease-carrying insects and animals into the United States," through "quarantine and immigration inspection for air travel."[32] As I will demonstrate in my discussion of *The Eternal Fight* (1948), the speed with which air travel could link dispersed locales established the cinematic map of transcontinental travel as an icon of the global spread of disease. The perceived threat that developing countries posed, via airplane, to the United States and Europe was summed up by the U.S. Surgeon General Hugh S. Cumming at a meeting of the Office International d'Hygiène Publique (OIHP) in Paris in 1930:

> The remarkable development of aerial transportation has brought with it international sanitary and public health problems of major importance. Regular lines of aircraft have been established, providing direct and rapid communication between areas in Africa, Asia, and South America, which have long been endemic centers of various pestilential diseases, such as cholera, plague, and yellow fever, and noninfected but infectible territory in Europe, North America, and in fact almost all the rest of the entire world. The journey by airplane from most of the endemic centers of these various pestilential diseases is usually less than the incubation period of these diseases, excepting journeys from endemic centers of cholera.[33]

This division of the globe into "infected" and "noninfected but infectible" continents drove the USPHS to undertake elaborate precautionary measures; the service attempted to halt contagions on a virtually microscopic level in a series of studies undertaken in 1931 "to determine the presence of insects, particularly [the malaria-carrying] *Aedes aegypti* mosquitoes, on aircraft arriving in the United States from tropical ports." The results of these investigations led to the spraying of pesticides (such as DDT) in airplane cabins prior to allowing passengers to disembark from the plane.[34]

While the advent of late-nineteenth-century communications technologies such as the telephone already seemed to create a dangerously rapid mode of transmitting invisible contagions—while nonetheless functioning as indispensable modern conveniences—the expansion of air travel prompted a further elaboration of the discursive formation in which global transportation networks signified as global disease networks.[35] However, despite the popular association of transportation and contagion, a confluence of events—cuts in public health funds after World War One, the 1921 and 1924 immigration acts, and the Depression of the 1930s—prevented the iconography of airborne contagion from significantly entering popular scientific media culture until after World War Two. But from the World War Two period onward, audiovisual production did radically expand, due largely to

the perceived urgency of combating the spread of invisible airborne contagions in the newly globalized project of world health.

(HOMO)SEXUAL CONTAGION AND MILITARY INVASION

The audiovisual discourse of world health enacts the compulsion to visualize
the invisible through its oscillation between indexical and artificial modes
of representation. While the medium of film would seem perfectly suited
to providing empirical evidence of the existence of invisible germs (and indeed, film *is* a privileged medium of representation for institutions of public health for precisely this reason), the impossibility of "documenting" the
spread of contagious disease inevitably leads to one of two displacements
(if not to both). The first of these slippages is the displacement of contamination onto visibly identifiable racial and sexual differences; the second is
the "capturing" of non-profilmic, animated images of contagion whose "authenticity" is affirmed by the equally artificial technique of voiceover. The
following analyses of *Hemolytic Streptococcus Control* and *The Eternal Fight*
include examples of both the indexical and the artificial poles of representation. In both films, invisible contagions threaten to penetrate the boundaries
of the human body, and this form of attack metonymically invokes national
invasion as well. Through this collapse, the hidden interior of the human
body becomes the site of a privileged form of national knowledge. However,
the camera cannot gain unmediated access to that interior corporeal truth
and, therefore, must invoke alternative means of constituting realism.

The United States Navy training film, *Hemolytic Streptococcus Control*
(1945), invokes the indexical pole to represent the sexualized transmission
of disease among male sailors, but as we will see, the failure of the indexical leads to the artificial representation of bodily and national contagions.
Within the homosocial navy, the bodily boundaries that might otherwise be
enforced through an insistence on gender heterogeneity threaten to break
down, thus casting suspicion on even the most mundane activities, such as
sharing a bottle of soda or washing windows. *Hemolytic Streptococcus Control*
instructs the intended audience of naval recruits on methods of preventing
the spread of contagious diseases that are caused by beta-hemolytic strepto-
cocci (such as scarlet fever, tonsillitis, bronchitis, and pneumonia). The story
of three shipmates who are all infected with the same germ, but whose symp-

toms are treated differently by the infirmary, is recounted through staged visual images and voiceover narration, with synchronized sound coming in only at the end of the film, when a naval officer directly addresses the camera to sum up the lessons learned. The disjuncture between image and sound in this film produces an (unintentionally) ironic distance between the "documentary" footage of naval activities and the authoritative voiceover, which interprets the meaning of the sailors' activities for the audience.[36] The soundtrack attempts to train the film's viewers in perceiving scenarios of contagion, by aurally identifying the disease-spreading activities occurring in sequences that might otherwise pass as representations of insignificant quotidian events, such as dishing out slices of pie or doing laundry. The voiceover thus serves the important—albeit unrecognized—function of explaining visual images that are meant to capture such unambiguous profilmic events as the spread of contagious disease.

The tension between visual and aural indexicality in this film is particularly interesting, considering that the presence of the voiceover as an interpretive guide is legitimized by the failure of the authority within the film—the medical doctor—accurately to interpret the signs of disease in the three infected sailors.[37] By allowing the medical professional's inadequacy to establish the primary narrative event of the film, *Hemolytic Streptococcus Control* admits the impossibility of successfully monitoring the spread of infectious disease in the public sphere. And yet, the alternative offered is an audiovisual representation of the invisible through a medium that must manipulate time (to provide a retrospective voiceover analysis) and space (to provide an animated vision of the spread of disease on local, regional, and national scales) to prove that contagion really is taking place, even if we cannot see or hear it happening. Cinema's ability to manipulate time and space has long been celebrated as one of the medium's unique attributes, but here this ability registers differently; on one hand, cinematic time and space *enable* representation of invisible contagions, on the other, recourse to such manipulations *undermines* the film's attempt to establish itself as empirical evidence of homosocial or sexual contagion.

As the film follows the different diagnosis and treatment of all three sailors, the inadequacy of the naked eye to detect the presence of communicable disease is revealed through the contrast between visual segments and voiceover. Visually, the opening sequence of the film presents a documentary-style reenactment of three sailors visiting sick bay, being examined by the doctor, and then being sent to the appropriate locations to recover from sickness or carry on with regular duties. All appears to be in order. However, the voiceover reveals what really happens (with the assistance of the film's melodramatic musical score):

> Three men went to sick call. The scarlet fever case was properly isolated. He will cause no trouble. The second man was admitted to the dispensary ward for a few days. While he is here, he will infect the other men in the ward. When he is released, he will infect the men in his barrack. This third man is sick, too. He will spread the germ to his shipmates. . . . Chances are good for an epidemic. This sick man not only infects his shipmates, but he contaminates everything he touches. Sweeping and bed-making re-suspend the dry bacteria and dust. Many men are thus exposed to hemolytic streptococcus, in small doses, over a prolonged period.

Thus, the truth underlying the images is not transparently available, but is only uncovered by a disembodied voice. Contagion in this film is thus revealed as a problem of homosocial contact; as the voiceover announces, some of the most dangerous sites of contagion are those places, "such as the dispensary and ship's service, where men intermingle." The paranoia regarding excessive closeness of male bodies to each other is repeated throughout the film, and this particular version of contagion anxiety is telling in a film produced as a navy training film.[38] The homosocial environment and the participation of the sailors in cooking and cleaning activities that are traditionally coded as feminine cast suspicion on the most fundamental elements of navy life. By offering isolation as the primary mode of preventing contagion, this film engages in the precise self-contradiction that drives the discourse of world health.

Consider the following segment. Several spaces occupied by large groups of men are represented, in a sequence of medium shots separated through horizontal wipes: first, we see men entering a room and sitting on benches, then milling around and waiting in line in the cafeteria, then sliding bunk beds across a room and sweeping around them, all in medium to medium-

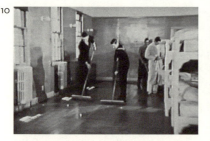

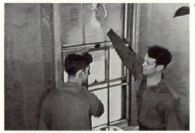

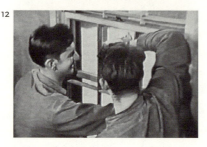

Hemolytic Streptococcus Control (1945)

long shots (figure 10). The next wipe cuts in to a high-angle medium close-up of two men washing a window, apparently talking and enjoying themselves, followed by a reverse shot, in close-up, showing one of the men laughing and then coughing (figures 11 and 12). This image dissolves into an animated sequence that begins with a representation of a room full of bunk beds, with an arrow leaping from bed to bed, leaving behind a trail that connects all of the bunks before the image dissolves into an aerial view of a row of buildings (presumably containing bunk beds), which are also linked by the same leaping arrow. Each sequential dissolve expands the visual perspective to take in more of the surrounding area as the arrow connects additional groups of buildings to each other, with the final dissolve revealing the arrow bounding across a map of the entire United States (figures 13–19). The voiceover during this sequence explains:

> Cleaning exercises allow men with different contagious diseases to come in close contact with each other. Those men, polishing the window, are just recovering from measles and scarlet fever. It is safe to predict that the boy with measles will soon be flat on his back with a streptococcal infection. An epidemic does explode, and it spreads—within the barrack,

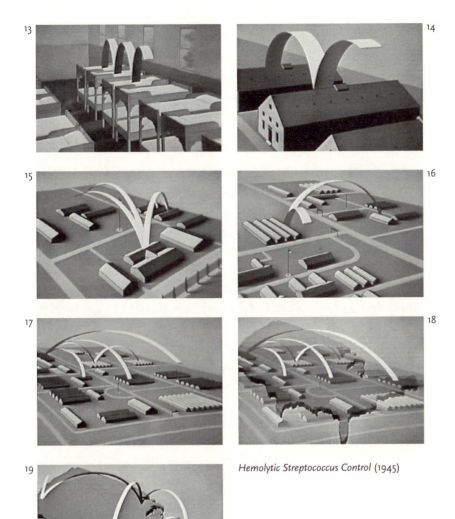

Hemolytic Streptococcus Control (1945)

barrack to barrack, from barracks to camp, camp to station, and station to station, all over the country.

Here we have two approaches to audiovisually representing invisible contagions—first, we have a voiceover that introduces a degree of discontinuity between the image and the soundtrack by interpreting seemingly innocent activities as incriminating, and then we have the animation, to reinforce the attribution of disease-spreading guilt to the window washers. The two modes of visualizing contagion are significantly linked through the implied threat of homosexuality, which the film suggests might result from two men sharing such traditionally feminine domestic chores. This link is literalized by the arrow leaping from bunk bed to bunk bed; thus homosociality becomes homosexuality, and this breakdown of bodily boundaries metonymically produces a nationwide epidemic. The film conceptualizes the individual body as the site of a privileged form of knowledge, not only by emphasizing the invisible germs that lurk inside of every body, but also by hyperbolizing (with the assistance of the maps) the scale of the potential contagions caused by an excessive proximity of male bodies to each other. The film's recourse to the authority of the disembodied voice and to animation indicates an implicit distrust of the authenticity of the image; the voiceover conveys the inadequacy of the visual image to "speak for itself," and the animation dispenses with the notion of capturing a profilmic indexical reality altogether. Such adamant refusal of film's ability to provide unmediated access to the "real" is striking in a genre that clearly embraces the scientific promise of technologies of visualization—particularly the microscope, X-rays, and cinema itself—and this refusal points to a pervasive hysteria in public health films about the simultaneous *impossibility* and absolute *necessity* of visualizing the invisible.

A similar contradiction informs the frequent appearance of national and global maps in these films. On one hand, abstracted images of geopolitical boundaries underscore the crucial definition of national identity through a public body that can securely maintain its own integrity against invasion. On the other hand, maps visualize the threat posed by "invisible enemies" that recognize *no* boundaries, thus entirely undermining the notion that the economic global hegemony of the postwar United States produces an exceptionalism that results in invulnerability to disease. The mapping sequences often invoke animation as they attempt to constitute realism through non-indexical means; the contradiction at the heart of the compulsion to visualize invisible contagions finds in animation a cinematic manipulation that affirms the authenticity of a map of disease by foregrounding the artifice of that very representation. While the discourse of contagion strives to make invisible germs visible in everyday life, the discourse founders in the medium that would seem most appropriately fitted to its aims; the potential for indexical representation of contagion on film must always be fulfilled through the nonindexical technique of animation.

The representation of contagion in the 1924 film *How Disease Is Spread* (discussed in the introduction) provides an interesting contrast with the postwar films, as the boundaries of contamination in the earlier film are securely contained within the borders of the United States—the notion of "world health" is off the map, so to speak. While the map of disease in *Hemolytic Streptococcus Control* also only reaches the borders of the United States, there are important historical differences in the vectors carrying contagion to those borders in each film. In *How Disease Is Spread*, an apparently white, middle-class woman spreads tuberculosis throughout the domestic sphere of consumer culture by participating in commercialized leisure activities; in *Hemolytic Streptococcus Control*, an apparently white naval serviceman spreads germs throughout the military forces charged with preventing invasion of u.s. borders, thus posing a threat to both physical and national bodies, by "intermingling" in excessive proximity with other men. The difference between the gender transgressions of the disease carrier in the 1924 film and the implied sexual transgressions in the 1945 film lies in the status of bodily boundaries in each. The discourse of world health is consistently concerned with the maintenance of bodily boundaries (both organic and national), the threat of penetration or dissolution of those boundaries, and the status of the body as a site of a privileged form of knowledge. As an axis of difference, sexuality necessarily draws attention to bodily borders in a way that gender may or may not; that is, sexual acts often involve contact between the inside and the outside of different bodies, and this form of border crossing has different implications than the gendered transgression of social boundaries, particularly concerning the spread of contagious disease.[39]

Moreover, as Michel Foucault has influentially argued, sexuality has been regarded as fundamentally constitutive of identity since the beginning of the nineteenth century, preempting every other axis of difference: "Causality in the subject, the unconscious of the subject, the truth of the subject in the other who knows, the knowledge he holds unbeknown to him, all this found an opportunity to deploy itself in the discourse of sex. Not, however, by reason of some natural property inherent in sex itself, but by virtue of the tactics of power immanent in this discourse."[40] The spread of disease through sexualized contact suggests a discursive conflation of invisible contagion with invisible sexuality; revelations of both are incessantly sought, and they are perceived as constituting privileged forms of knowledge. Thus, the emphasis on gender in the 1924 film is not linked to the power/knowledge system that underlies the discourse of world health, while the national map in the postwar film is endowed with a new discursive significance as globalization becomes an explicit—and prominent—feature of the postwar public health discourse linking contagion with identity.

RACIAL CONTAGION AND GLOBAL COMMUNICATION

The threat of contagious disease expands to encompass the entire globe in *The Eternal Fight*, a film produced for the United Nations Film Board in 1948. In this film, the sources of contagious disease are identified with specific national sources outside of the United States, but their location beyond American borders nonetheless threatens those within the nation's bounds. Like *Hemolytic Streptococcus Control* and *How Disease Is Spread*, this film combines a fictionalized account of the spread of a particular disease (in this case, typhus—black plague, carried by an unwitting sailor), with a discussion of the ease with which diseases can be spread around the globe, specifically because of their invisibility.

The film begins by tracing the history of medical progress in the "eternal fight" against contagious disease, intercutting historical reenactments of scientific discoveries (such as Louis Pasteur's discovery "that microbes were at the root of contagious diseases") with images of a map of western Europe and North America that situates each discovery in relation to the next. Once the account reaches the period of the Industrial Revolution, reenactments are replaced with documentary footage of factories spewing smoke, steelworkers pouring molten ore, and textile mills with rooms packed full of women at sewing machines. At this point, the progress narrative shifts to a narrative of decline; despite the advances of modern communication and transportation technologies, the primary feature of the postindustrial era is epidemic disease. As the melodramatic voiceover announces, "Men, women and children, crowded into cities, became part of a vast machine. Deprived of sun and the fresh nourishment of the country, men's bodies rusted, became more vulnerable to contagion." Here, as in the film discussed above, neither the indexical image nor the interpretive voiceover can capture the full impact of contagion on a global scale, and thus the film turns to animation.

Beginning with a close-up of a stylized locomotive wheel, the voiceover announces, "New means of transportation brought the world tight and close together, making it one tremendous and congested city." Meanwhile, the animated perspective tracks back to reveal the whole train, and then cuts away to an aerial view of the train's path, departing from an abstracted city, represented by a chaotic jumble of crisscrossed lines. This contrast between urban and rural parallels the broader dichotomy between modern and premodern, First and Third Worlds, that forms the foundation of the discourse of world health. Suddenly, a giant skull appears superimposed above the city grid, as the train charges through the countryside, represented by a landscape of mountains and hills (figure 20). Along the train's path a giant hourglass appears, signaling the collapse of time and space inaugurated by such products of the industrial revolution as the locomotive, the airplane, and, of course, the motion picture (figures 21 and 22).[41] Accompanied by a suspenseful, race-against-the-clock musical score, the voiceover explains, "From a disease-infected zone, the traveler now became, unwittingly, a carrier of deadly germs. Wherever he went, the germs stayed, and spread." When the train reaches the next city grid, it leaves in its path a mark which expands to become a giant black cross towering over the city, with "CHOLERA!!" in bold letters beside it (figures 23 and 24). Meanwhile, the camera pans left to the far edge of the city, where a ship departs, and, upon reaching the opposite shore, a gray area of infection spreads over the city from the port: "Epidemics break out, far from the known infected areas. Country to country, continent to continent, the deadly cargo of microbes is transported, menacing on a vast scale the very existence of humanity" (figures 25–27).

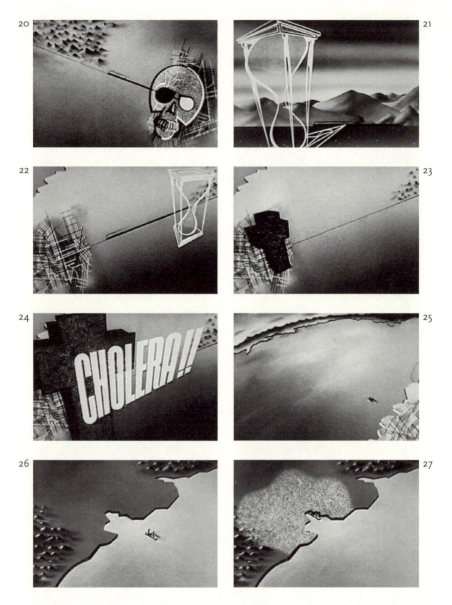

The Eternal Fight (1948)

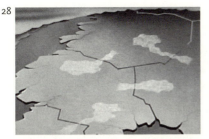

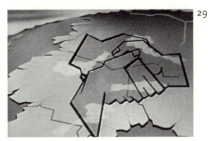

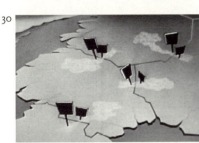

The Eternal Fight (1948)

Here, the supposed benefits of modernization that demarcate the bound-aries between "developed" and "underdeveloped" countries are themselves identified as the vectors of contagion. Furthermore, although the techno-logically produced collapse of space and time is represented as a distinctive feature of modernity, occupants of the spatio-temporally distant realm of premodernity—or what Anne McClintock has called "anachronistic space" —are nonetheless vulnerable to the rapid spread of contagion associated with modern life.[42] Over a montage of animated newspaper headlines in vari-ous languages, the voiceover proclaims, "Mass infection and epidemics are a threat to every city, to every nation. Scientific and medical work on a local scale are no longer enough. Thus, in common defense, nations join in inter-national agreement in the battle against epidemics." Here, over a geographi-cal mass divided by three national boundary lines, are superimposed three giant hands, shaking in agreement (figures 28 and 29). Along each side of the borders, signposts appear, apparently intended to prevent contagious dis-eases from entering noninfected national territories (figure 30).

Although it is not mentioned by name here, in the preceding sequence this international health surveillance handshake is clearly identified as an accomplishment of the League of Nations. But this confident success at constructing international boundaries against contagion is soon undermined by a segment on World War Two and the bodily ravages that it brings. Now the animation is replaced by documentary footage of war-torn Europe, and the global contagion represented in the earlier animated sequence is repeated through a live-action dramatization of an individual sailor who unwittingly carries black plague. Unlike the first animated contagion sequence, this later episode places equal emphasis on the role of transportation *and* communication technologies in both enabling and preventing the spread of disease.

As the sequence opens, the voiceover laments the difficulties of life as a sailor, especially when the call to ship out coincides with one's wife being stricken by illness. In classic melodramatic form, the sailor embraces his wife (to a weepy soundtrack) as she lays suffering in bed in their dismal, threadbare flat. As he kisses her, the camera pans left to reveal the source of the ailment: a dead rat laying in a corner of the kitchen floor. From the sailor's departure we cut to a close-up of the feverish wife, and tracking back, find that an ellipsis has occurred—she is now in the hospital, and having diagnosed plague, the examining doctor rapidly retreats from the room, destroys his scrubs, and moves immediately to the telephone. A montage of transnational telecommunications efficiency distinguishes this outbreak from the animated cholera outbreak earlier in the film; while the previous epidemic was caused by unregulated technological development, the current epidemic is contained by parallel technological advances put to good use. As the international health surveillance machinery moves into gear, the infected sailor lays quivering on a cot aboard the ship, until the Quarantine Service of the USPHS comes aboard to bring the sick man ashore, inoculate the rest of the crew, and fumigate the ship with cyanide gas.

But the successful detection of contagious disease aboard a slow-moving ship is not sufficient evidence that global health surveillance mechanisms can indeed halt the spread of disease; the crucial test is in the regulation of air travel, with its potential for traversing national and continental borders in a matter of hours (figures 31–33). The narrator describes the postwar collapse of space and time, over a montage of airplane passengers disembarking: "Today there are no distances. Today aeroplanes link continents as trains link cities. Today the peoples of the world are one people, joined by wings over the globe. Today people of all races, of every level, move from country

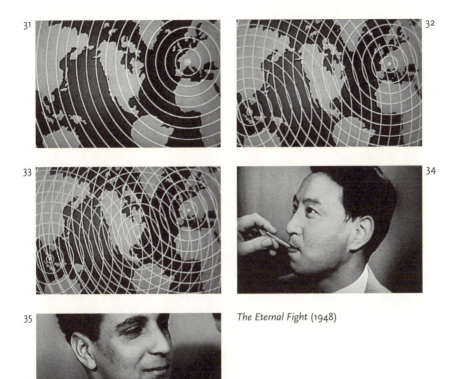

The Eternal Fight (1948)

to country in a matter of hours." Significantly, at this point in the film the montage shifts from images of airplanes to images of different ethnic groups undergoing medical examinations (figures 34 and 35). The problem of global contagions is thus collapsed onto the "problem" of racial difference at the moment when the film focuses in on the most vulnerable points of national and bodily border penetration: the airports. Accompanied by a montage of regulatory mechanisms for transportation and communication technologies such as customs inspections and airplane schedule boards, the voiceover articulates the anxiety that drives the discourse of world health: "Today vital medical control is established around the modern points of international exchange: the airports. The network of health information and services has

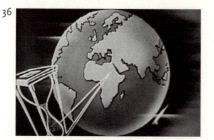

36

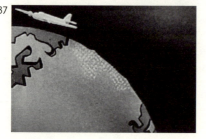

37

The Eternal Fight (1948)

been extended here from the seaport organization. But is this sufficient? How long can it take before a potential epidemic is detected?"

At this moment, the characteristic failure of the compulsion to visually represent invisible contagions appears yet again. The answer to the narrator's question is expressed not through an empirically grounded epidemiological map, but through an animated airplane orbiting the globe, with a giant hourglass emerging from Africa and marking the origins of a contagious disease whose spread is facilitated by the airplane flying overhead, then sprinkling particles of African infection over southeast Asia as it passes (figures 36 and 37). The narration repeats the worry expressed by the u.s. surgeon general in 1930: "From one continent to another, only a few hours' flying time. But cholera takes longer to show itself. And yellow fever: three to six days. And the incubation period of smallpox: from seven to sixteen days." At this point, the animation links up with filmed images of potential disease carriers, sitting innocently on an airplane. By intercutting the animated map of contagion and the indexical images of disease carriers, the invisibility of contagion is at once affirmed and denied; it is through the juxtaposition of profilmic "reality" with manipulations of that reality (voiceover and animation) that disease is articulated to the physical bodies that traverse geopolitical borders.

Significantly, even the voiceover acknowledges the contradiction under-lying the attempt to regulate world health:

> Passengers in a modern plane look perfectly healthy. They are. But how do we know? That little girl—when she got the doll did she receive germs as well? Some passengers may be germ carriers, perhaps already in the incubation stage. They'll reach their destinations before any symp-toms show. The Quarantine Service can't keep every plane and passenger grounded for several days to effect thorough medical control. Today that system of defense is no longer enough. Today epidemics must be crushed at the very source.

But once the problem of invisible contagion is admitted, it is immediately answered by a further specification of the collapse between national and physical borders: invisibility is made visible through signifiers of national and ethnic identity. The emphasis on national borders in this sequence is paired with images of personified national identities, thus producing con-crete visual associations between racial and ethnic difference and the threat of invisible contagions that could emanate from those differently marked bodies.

When we return to the animated globe, infection sprinkles are now visi-ble in India, Africa, the Middle East, and southeast Asia. The boundaries between "infected" and "noninfected but infectible" zones are now clearly delineated, as the camera zooms in on an arrow arcing from India to west-ern Europe and depositing disease sprinkles there (figures 38 and 39). The balance of geopolitical power is now recognized as a vital component in global health surveillance, as is the contradiction that globalization is both cause and potential cure of transnational contagions: "Unfortunately, in some countries, contagious diseases exist in an endemic state—that is, per-manently. India, for instance, has certain areas that are always infected with cholera. This plague can extend to western Europe." As in *How Disease Is Spread* and *Hemolytic Streptococcus Control*, the paths of contagion are re-peatedly represented here, until the entire globe is covered, even the United States, as an arrow reaches over from southeast Asia: "And cholera in Japan could strike suddenly at the West coast of the United States" (figure 40). This boundary crossing finally elicits some response, and a giant "X" appears

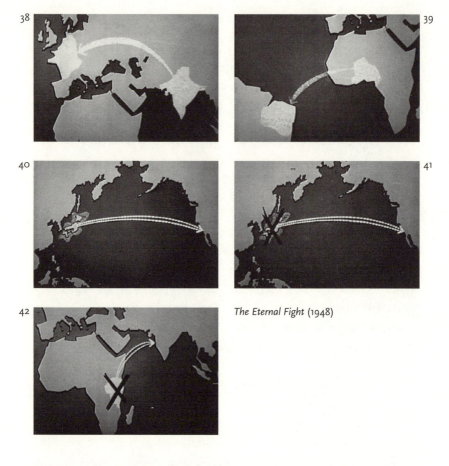

38 39

40 41

42   *The Eternal Fight* (1948)

over Japan, eliminating both the contagion and its national source (figures 41 and 42).[43]

It is the recognition of globalization as a fundamental and self-contradictory element in the discourse of contagion that leads to the film's consolidation of artificial and indexical representations of disease, in the form of nationally and racially marked bodies as the objects of the World Health Organization. The voiceover sums up the postwar situation, over an image of the globe in which all land masses are infected, and a giant skull covers the entire planet: "Permanently infected zones are localized, but may cover large areas of territory, sometimes entire continents. Modern transportation poses new dangers of complete universal contagion. The struggle against epidemics is a global one, for the danger of death is worldwide."

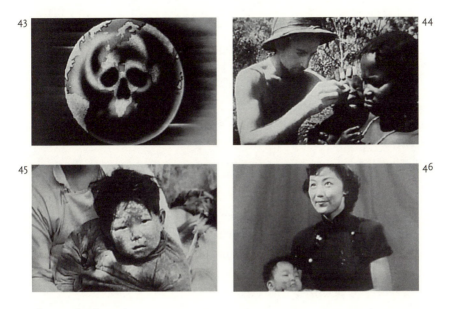

43 44

45 46

The Eternal Fight (1948)

The skull is replaced with a question mark, as the narrator asks, "Then, what is the answer?" (figure 43). The response: an image of United Nations pamphlets, accompanied by triumphant music. "Within the framework of the United Nations, a new organization exists to promote the welfare of all people: the World Health Organization. . . . The prime objective of the World Health Organization is the fight against disease, on a global scale." This grand statement of the solution to "universal contagion" leads to documentary footage of medical scenarios in which white doctors treat nonwhite patients in developing countries, and through this montage of contagion and vaccination, nationally and racially marked bodies function as indexical, transparently legible surfaces that signify an interior corporeal truth: that the essence of these bodies is disease (figures 44–46). This collapse not only affirms the racial difference between contaminated bodies and their imperial others, but also affirms that, despite the film's reliance on animation and voiceover throughout, documentary footage *can* visually represent the invisible. Even if the body captured on film is only legible when subjected to extrafilmic manipulations, it is nonetheless indistinguishable in its materiality. It is precisely through their self-contradictory reliance on this form of indexical realism that the public health films under investigation here assert their own objectivity. By maintaining that racial and sexual difference transparently correlate to contagion, postwar films such as *Hemolytic Streptococcus Control* and *The Eternal Fight* establish their own ideological structures of signification as universal truths and, thus, as authentic documents of realism.

CONCLUSION

In the postwar audiovisual discourse of world health, the linkage of external bodily difference with hidden internal dangers is established through the insistence on locating the sources of individual contagions, despite the simultaneous recognition that, since the advent of modern transportation technologies, diseases have continually circled the globe and thus cannot be pinpointed as originating in a specific time and place. By moving from a paranoia so generalized that it even casts aspersions on a little girl's doll to a paranoia quite explicitly based on sources in the so-called Third World, *The Eternal Fight* highlights the hysteria about globalization that informs the discourse of world health. On one hand, this discourse celebrates the ideals of Western civilization, in terms of bureaucratic rationalization, medical and scientific progress, and democracy, and these achievements are promoted as the justification and mandate for the spread of United States global hegemony. On the other hand, this discourse views any international contact as the site of a breakdown of boundaries that will inevitably result in worldwide contagion. This contradiction is repeated at the level of representation through an adamant disavowal of any one-to-one relationship between visual images and the "real" and through a simultaneous avowal of the possibility of representing the real through increasing levels of manipulation of the relationship between image and sound—that is, through voiceover and animation. In other words, the adamant insistence on the possibility of documenting contagion can meet with success only through the use of entirely "nondocumentary" modes of representation. And it is this tension— between the pursuit of an indexical image of contagion and the denial of the existence of that image—that provides the foundation for the concept of "world health," with its paranoid fantasy of maintaining organic and national boundaries that are continually threatening to dissolve.

These physical and geopolitical boundaries parallel the technological boundary that has separated images and sounds since the invention of cinema, not only during the silent era, but also after the development of synchronized sound. This feature is clearly not unique to the public health films under investigation here, but the ideological implications of the image/ sound split resonate in both Hollywood and public health cinemas. Indeed, the classical Hollywood style of "transparent" editing, which is based on elaborate manipulations of images and sounds, is meant to produce the illusion that the two sources are *not* severed.[44] The efforts required to secure the apparent unity of image and sound in many ways delimit the boundaries of the classical Hollywood mode of representation, which has become so ubiquitous as to define the commonplace view of "realistic" representation.[45] Moreover, the imaginary unity of image and sound so characterizes the globally dominant classical Hollywood style that counter-cinemas often establish their opposition to the imperialism of u.s. visual culture by insisting upon a disjunction between images and sounds as a means of foregrounding the artifice of what usually passes as a hegemonic definition of realism.[46] This version of realism has ideological implications on geopolitical and subjective levels; not only has the economic dominance of the Hollywood film industry monopolized theatrical exhibition in the United States and abroad, to the detriment of indigenous, independent productions, but also the content (and subsequent political positioning) of Hollywood films has elicited a very specific kind of spectator with a very particular worldview.[47] As Mary Ann Doane has argued, this subject position implies a certain relation to the status of the body in defining one's sense of self, and the satisfaction afforded by Hollywood's favored construction of subjectivity depends upon the unity of image and sound in filmic constructions of reality:

> The body reconstituted by the technology and practices of the cinema is a *phantasmatic* body, which offers a support as well as a point of identification for the subject addressed by the film. . . . The attributes of this phantasmatic body are first and foremost unity (through an emphasis on a coherence of the senses) and presence-to-itself. The addition of sound to the cinema introduces the possibility of representing a fuller (and organically unified) body.[48]

Thus, the existence of a clearly marked gap between the audio and the visual is often read as a sign of a given film's resistance to the classical Hollywood aim of interpellating a coherent, self-present, unified subject (implicitly white, male, heterosexual, propertied, literate, and so forth) as the ideal spectator of its films. What is interesting about the movement between realist audiovisual unification and antirealist divorcement of the audio from the visual in postwar public health films is that this fluctuation belies a profound ambivalence about the desirability, to say nothing of the attainability, of a coherent subjectivity founded upon an imagined unity of the physical body with its subjective image. Such ambivalence is striking in a discourse that is founded in the postwar celebration of u.s. global hegemony, which articulates the ideals of world health through the binary opposition of normative healthy, white, Western masculinity to all "others."

The oscillation between the indexical and the artificial modes of representing invisible contagions points to a pervasive schizophrenia in public health films, about the simultaneous impossibility and absolute necessity of visualizing the invisible. As argued above, this documentary/nondocumentary dialectic provides the representational foundation of a discourse that attains cultural dominance during the course of the twentieth century (and particularly in the postwar period)—namely, the world health and epidemiological discourse on the relationship between modernization and global sanitation—that structures the process by which audiovisual technologies of information produce knowledge about bodies and power. The concept of "world health" collapses discourses of globalization onto discourses of bodily integrity, thus producing a highly self-contradictory epistemological formation that is preoccupied with the borders of physical bodies as signifiers of national geographies. Even while globalization is celebrated as the source of prosperity for the "Third World," it is also blamed as the source of transnational contagions. And even as audiovisual technologies are celebrated as media that will enable universal communication, they are revealed to be failures at capturing unmediated images of "the real." The audiovisual discourse of world health hysterically and compulsively undermines its own attempts to prove the ontological veracity of the image: the impossibility of seeing contagion results in the proliferation of images of disease.

CHAPTER 3

From Inner to Outer Space:
WORLD HEALTH AND THE POSTWAR ALIEN INVASION FILM

Tropical parasites causing disease seem unrelated to the everyday living
of most Americans, but two things—World War II and global travel—
have brought them together.

R. C. WILLIAMS, *The United States Public Health Service*

PUBLIC HEALTH AND SCIENCE FICTION

The public health crisis provoked by the spread of anthrax through the U.S.
postal system in fall 2001 was compounded by a representational crisis that
plagued mass media depictions of the spread of contagion. The threat of contamination by invisible spores of the deadly bacteria rapidly seemed to become universal as the symbolic function of the primary targets (news media
and politicians) was radically democratized by the simple fact that almost
everyone in the country receives mail. This sense of omnipresence was exacerbated by the fact that the familiar conventions for saturation coverage
of a national crisis failed in the face of the invisible threat. Unlike the in-
tensely graphic and seemingly endless loop imagery of the twin towers collapsing the previous month, the appearance and potential spread of anthrax
utterly lacked an arresting visual image. But just as the invisibility of anthrax
prompted emergency containment procedures on the part of public health
personnel (who searched frantically to locate new and residual sites of infection), the absence of a clearly identifiable iconography of anthrax drove the
news media to undertake their own (unsuccessful) search for easily repro-
ducible signs of contagion.

This anxious search for imagery of contagion has often troubled the pro-
ponents of public health education. As earlier chapters have demonstrated,
the field of public health has a long history of associating visual represen-

tation of a disease with successful prevention of the spread of that disease. For this reason, audiovisual media have played a crucial role in information campaigns aimed at containing outbreaks of communicable disease. However, as in the case of anthrax, the representations of other biological threats have also failed at documenting the moment of contagion; the invisibility of the process of contamination always requires a displacement of the bacterium (or virus) onto its more tangible, and thus more visually representable vectors. Historically, this displacement has often entailed attaching disease to images of racial and sexual "deviance," as AIDS was initially represented in the early 1980s through racialized African or Haitian bodies and sexualized gay white male bodies.

As scholars Jasbir Puar and Amit Rai argued in an essay on 9/11, the representation of the Middle Eastern terrorist draws upon historical images of "monsters and fags" whose bodies are seen as containing hidden contaminations that are understood as primarily ideological, but which implicitly connote a linkage of Islamic extremism with deviant sexual and racial identity.[1] What their essay does not address is the interconnection between this form of bodily pathology and the threat of invisible contamination that it carries. The slippage in television news media coverage from the search for the source of the anthrax attacks to the search for Osama Bin Laden reveals the deep anxiety that has long motivated the pursuit of world health: the fear that a terrorist (or some other deadly contagion) is hidden inside of every immigrant to the United States. As we will see, the recent expressions of this anxiety draw heavily upon an iconography developed half a century earlier, in response to fears of a different sort of invisible invader.

Since the 1980s, the global proliferation of varied biological and electronic viruses has dominated the daily news with a frequency that suggests a world on the brink of apocalyptic crisis. In these reports, the dissolution of national borders that is said to characterize the supposedly new global economy is often represented as an effect of the "new media" that—in combination with the international movement of finance, labor, and commodities—links even the farthest reaches of the globe in a virtual web, with alternately democratizing and contaminating results. But the rhetoric of contagion that pervades the contemporary discourse of globalization has a much longer history than these panicked reports would suggest, and in this chapter, I examine one key articulation of this history through the genre of American science fiction film in the 1950s.

In this period, health and hygiene were seen as integral to Cold War nation-building campaigns, especially in opposition to the strict and vigorous appearance of the Soviet Union's Communist youth. The concern with physical fitness had been a national issue since the practice of public health was institutionalized in the 1930s, but the linkage of national identity with healthy bodies dates back even further—to the formative years of the republic. From the Sanitary Commission formed during the Civil War to the fight against yellow fever during the Spanish American War and the influenza pandemic of World War One, public health and national security have been discursively and logistically connected. The prominent role of the USPHS in fighting the 1918 influenza pandemic popularized this linkage, but it wasn't until the generally poor physical fitness of American troops seemed to threaten defeat during World War Two that the institution took on the role of promoting a national ideal of physical fitness—an ideal that is captured in both public health and Hollywood films. The increasing involvement of the USPHS in different realms of social life, combined with the new medical techniques and antibiotics developed during the war, led to greatly enhanced social prestige for the fields of medicine and public health in postwar American culture.[2] The increasing prominence of institutions of public health, and the proliferation of audiovisual technologies in daily life (such as the expanded use of films and filmstrips in education and industry after World War Two, not to mention the new availability of television) combined to disseminate the imagery of world health throughout popular culture.[3]

However, a history of public health in this period based solely on cinematic representations would lead viewers to draw some strikingly erroneous conclusions. In fact, a comparison of cinematic and written accounts of the 1950s reveals a telling contradiction. The development of antibiotics during the postwar period transformed the treatment of communicable diseases, leading to optimistic declarations that venereal and other contagions had been effectively conquered by penicillin. While such proclamations proved far from accurate, they nonetheless drove public health policy away from its focus on contagious disease, shifting emphasis toward chronic diseases such as cancer.[4] However, this shift is not reflected in the films produced in the postwar period; on the contrary, these films are almost obsessively concerned with the consequences of globalization for accomplishing the ideals of "world health," and this focus frames the very definition of "health" in terms of constructing and maintaining boundaries against contagious, not chronic disease. Moreover, the history of Hollywood film production in this period reveals an intense fascination with processes of contagion, especially in the popular genre of science fiction. In these films, national and physical bodies are invaded by foreign agents that destroy individual and social integrity and consequently threaten both national and international security.

The absence of a direct parallel between the institutional history of public health and the cinematic self-representation of its institutions demonstrates that motion pictures cannot be viewed as transparent windows onto the past. That is, instead of reflecting the shift toward funding and investigating chronic diseases, the public health films produced in this period reveal a different set of concerns that express their complex relationship to contemporaneous events in public health. While it might seem obvious that motion pictures, like all cultural and artistic productions, are mediated by the partial and subjective (rather than universal and objective) perspectives of their producers, the scholarship on the postwar period has nonetheless tended quite consistently toward the transparent reflection model of analysis. Precisely because of this common misapprehension of the relationship between film and history, the cinematic preoccupation with contagious disease in the 1950s provides an important occasion for considering how both scientific and popular representations construct meaning in and about the public sphere.[5] To explore these interconnections, this chapter will compare the modes of representing infection in public health and Hollywood films. For, just as the public health films do not clearly convey postwar health policy, the science fiction films that I discuss do not simply reflect the widespread paranoia about Communism that is often assumed to explain all aspects of Cold War American culture. While the threat of Communism was undoubtedly a crucial component of the postwar social imaginary, the language of anti-Communism was itself entwined with the cultural discourse of world health.[6] With its rhetoric of invasion by invisible enemies who spread the ideology of Communism like a highly infectious contagion, the language of anti-Communism was heavily influenced by the imagery and anxieties of world health.[7]

I argued in chapters 1 and 2 that the central aim of postwar public health films was to visually represent invisible contagions and that the specific modes of representing disease were institutionally aligned with educational, not entertainment cinema as a result of the debates over film regulation in the 1930s. In this chapter I demonstrate that although the two film genres were officially separated, the discourse of world health pervaded both public health and Hollywood films in the postwar period. The stylistic intersections between scientific and popular cultural forms also reveal an ideological over-lap: the ability to visually represent the invisible amounts to the ability to prevent the invasion of national and bodily boundaries, whether by foreign diseases or extraterrestrial aliens. The Hollywood mode of representing national boundaries under siege shares in the view of world health as a system that polices the boundaries of nation-states and continents across whose borders contagions threaten to spread. And through the imagery of physical and national border invasion, public health and science fiction films reveal their shared anxieties about the effects of globalization. Moreover, the concern in both genres with visibility and invisibility highlights the permeability of generic boundaries between educational and entertainment cinemas, thus explaining the absorption of world health iconography into popular culture. The similarities between narrative fiction films and instructional nonfiction films appear particularly significant when considered in light of the institutionalized elimination of public health themes from entertainment cinema that resulted from the revision of the Production Code in 1934. Despite formal regulations separating the production, distribution, and exhibition of public health and science fiction films, both sets of films are driven by a desire to visually represent the invisible interior of the body. This cross-generic stylistic cohesion is a testament to the cultural pervasiveness of the ideology of world health.

INDEXICAL AND ARTIFICIAL, STOCK FOOTAGE AND SPECIAL EFFECTS

The preoccupation with the boundaries of visibility that characterizes post-war public health films also defines postwar Hollywood cinema, especially the emergent genre of science fiction. The popularity of the genre in the 1950s is crucially linked to the expansion of image-based culture in the postwar United States, and as the genre proliferates, popular culture becomes increasingly permeated by the imagery of world health.[8] As I argued in earlier chapters, competing versions of realism underlie the dialectic of visibility and invisibility, alternately relying on indexical images of racially and sexually marked bodies and artificially animated maps of contagion. This contradictory but nonetheless foundational drive toward realism links the postwar public health and Hollywood films that articulate the ideals of world health. In fact, the film that is most often cited as the inauguration of the science fiction film genre, *Destination Moon* (1950), is almost invariably described in terms of its realism and documentary feel: "A quasi documentary such as *Destination Moon* (Irving Pichel, 1950), was an attempt to give a realistic picture of what the first moon landing might involve."[9] The film's use of documentary-style stock footage at key narrative moments establishes a convention that will pervade science fiction throughout its golden age in the 1950s.[10] In addition to its privileging of "the real" through documentary footage, *Destination Moon* also invokes animation at another key narrative moment; thus, the film's alternation between indexicality and artificiality merits brief discussion here.[11]

Opening with a failed rocket launch that is suspected of being the result of sabotage, *Destination Moon* is the story of the aerospace industry's peacetime mobilization to construct and launch a rocket to the moon, in the name of national defense. Explaining that the federal government will eventually turn to the private sector for assistance, and that preparedness isn't just for wartime, Army General Thayer convinces James Barnes, of Barnes Aircraft Corporation, to use his factory for the construction of a new rocket. These two, in turn, must convince the captains of American industry to invest in the project, and the resulting sequence exemplifies the oscillation between indexicality and artificiality that characterizes the intersection of science fiction and public health.

Barnes and Thayer call together the wealthiest businessmen in the nation (all dressed in tuxedos and gathered in a formally appointed clubhouse setting) to pitch the rocketship project to them. In the middle of this pivotal scene, in which the fate of the rocket (and therefore the fate of the film's narrative development) will be decided, the proposal is turned over to an audiovisual aid—specifically, an animated film—"prepared especially for this meeting." In the midst of *Destination Moon*, a "realist" film whose tone resembles nothing so much as an illustrated lecture, this cartoon serves the same function that it would in an educational public health film, alternating between direct address lectures, "indexical" documentary footage, and "artificially" animated maps of contagion.[12] The film, starring the popular children's cartoon character Woody Woodpecker, collapses its own diegetic world with that of *Destination Moon* through a form of direct address that enacts the slippage between fantasy and reality that pervades the discourse of world health. The animated protagonist (an anthropomorphized bird) begins the film within the film in the subjective position of a dubious investor, scoffing at the idea of a rocket to the moon, calling it "ridiculous, comic book stuff." The conventionalized omniscient and omnipotent human narrator and sketch artist within the cartoon intervenes at this point, showing Woody Woodpecker the covers of *Life* magazine, *Look*, *Pic*, *Collier's*, and a number of the "biggest daily newspapers," to prove that mass culture in America supports and believes in the possibility that a rocket could indeed reach the moon.[13] Woody becomes interested and examines one of the magazine articles—itself also titled "Destination Moon"—more closely. The remainder of the cartoon is spent dispelling the notion that it is impossible for a vessel without wings or propellers to fly, and, once convinced, Woody Woodpecker offers his own $2 donation, asking "When do we start building?" The audience within the film applauds, and Barnes repeats the question: "Gentlemen, when *do* we start building?"

At this point, the general steps in, shifting the rhetorical tone from entertainment to education and recasting the relevance of the project in geopolitical terms: "There is absolutely no way to stop an attack from outer space. The first country that can use the moon for the launching of missiles will control the earth. That, gentlemen, is the most important military fact of this century." The philanthropic capitalists eagerly support the project, and their applause dissolves into a documentary-style construction sequence that effectively collapses the indexical and the artificial, the stock footage and the special effects. Or, in the terms of film scholar Adam Knee's analysis, the sequence collapses the fantastic with the scientific:

The near-documentary style detail with which the film pursues its subject of lunar travel helped establish a convention which long continued to resurface in science fiction films—a sense not only that the narrative is extrapolated from currently verifiable scientific fact, but that the film is itself a kind of document of astounding events, a rendering plausible of the fantastic. This documentary thrust can be seen, for example, in regular appearances of stock newsreel footage of battles and of rocket blasts throughout films of the genre in the 1950s. Not only does the use of this footage become a common generic convention, but certain documentary images are repeated with such frequency as to gain an iconographic weight in and of themselves. Paradoxically, and significantly, it is often in the films' fantastic special effects sequences that stock actuality footage becomes most central: through montage, presently known realities of war or of rocket experimentation literally become part of the fantastic, recast into the image of an extrapolated near-future.[14]

As I argued in previous chapters, this "paradoxical" contrast between special effects and stock actuality sequences is in fact not paradoxical at all, though it is certainly a striking representational technique. The dialectic of indexicality and artificiality may be self-contradictory, but it develops and proceeds according to the consistent overarching logic of world health.

An additional linkage occurs at the iconographic level: the UN, and even more significantly, the World Health Organization (WHO), had been so rapidly assimilated into the postwar social imaginary that by simply invoking these institutions, a film could immediately frame its particular disaster in the context of scientific realism and globalization. Susan Sontag recognized this convention in her essay on science fiction cinema, "The Imagination of Disaster." Summarizing what she sees as the three variations on the generic script of the science fiction film, Sontag points to a narrative phase:

> In the capital of the country, conferences between scientists and the military take place, with the hero lecturing before a chart, map, or blackboard. A national emergency is declared. Reports of further destruction. Authorities from other countries arrive in black limousines. All international tensions are suspended in view of the planetary emergency. This stage often includes a rapid montage of news broadcasts in various lan-

guages, a meeting at the UN, and more conferences between the military and the scientists. Plans are made for destroying the enemy.[15]

Sontag argues that science fiction cinema addresses two parallel fears that characterize postwar life: the fear of banality (the homogenization effect of mass culture), and the fear of annihilation (by nuclear war). The oft-cited themes of conformity and nuclear or Communist anxiety are clearly central for understanding postwar American culture, and yet they fail to recognize the specific techniques and discourses of visuality that define not only cinematic representations but, increasingly, most institutions of daily life in the "information age." (In fact, the technologies of representation, information, and transportation play a crucial role in defining the imagery of contagious globalization in this period.) Nonetheless, Sontag's recognition of the iconographic status of the UN and, by extension, of the WHO has important implications for my argument here.

For instance, in the opening scenes of *Them!*, a 1954 film about the invasion of the United States by giant, atomically altered ants, a radio broadcast contrasts the postwar faith in medical progress with the unraveling narrative of nature out of control.[16] In a ransacked general store, amid a desert windstorm in the American Southwest, an unattended radio fades in and out on the soundtrack, reporting "elsewhere, from Geneva, Switzerland, comes heartening word of new strides in the field of medicine. Dr. Adolf Renselier, addressing members of the World Health Organization, now convening in that city, declares that diseases such as malaria, cholera, and sleeping sickness have been entirely wiped out from areas that formerly were in a state approximating permanent. . . ." The visual images accompanying this announcement show not only the inexplicable destruction of the small building, but also a dead body laying in the basement. When the radio fades back in, we hear "still a closely guarded secret." In a sequence that sets the tone of the film to follow, the invocation of the WHO serves to establish the contradictions of postwar prosperity (leading to international control over the spread of disease) and chaos (the reality that global sanitation may be declared to be winning, but such victory is in fact impossible). At the end of this sequence, a policeman is killed offscreen by a giant ant. The juxtaposition of the WHO's optimistic declarations with the reality that man is losing the battle

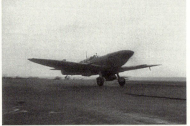

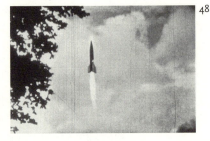

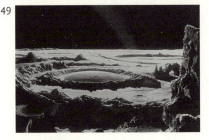

War of the Worlds (1953)

with nature demonstrates the WHO's symbolic importance to postwar political and popular cultures and reveals the contradictions that define the project of world health.

Moreover, by framing the dialectic of visibility and invisibility in the context of globalization, science fiction cinema reinforces the linkage of national and bodily invasion with world health, as a brief overview of *The War of the Worlds* (1953) will demonstrate.[17] The film opens with stock documentary footage of World Wars One and Two, presented through a newsreel-style montage and voiceover that contextualizes the third world war within the mass-mediated archive of twentieth-century history (figures 47 and 48). Cutting from the journalistic opening to a rapid credits sequence, the film recommences at the opposite pole of realism; an animated sequence displays the different planets in Earth's solar system, and a voiceover explains that the Martians are invading Earth in search of an atmosphere suitable to their survival (figure 49). The oscillation between the indexical and the artificial is particularly striking due to the film's efforts to ensure its own reception as an authentic documentation of "the real" through the newsreel framing device, which is reasserted throughout the film via intermittent voiceover announcements that serve as plot exposition.[18]

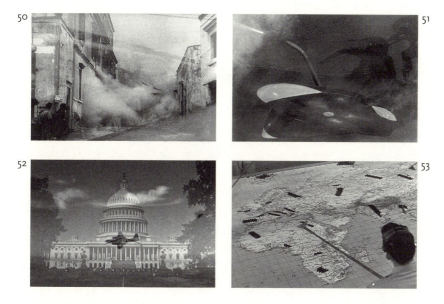

War of the Worlds (1953)

Alternating between documentary footage of war and special effects of alien spacecraft, this film performs the same oscillation between celebrating and condemning globalization that most postwar public health films enact (figures 50–53). By the end of the film, the alien destruction of earth, which has been sensationally represented through stock war and natural disaster footage, seems inevitable—all but two of the main characters have been killed off, and the romantic couple has been separated. Almost all hope is lost, when the deus ex machina—contagious disease—comes in. The destruction unexpectedly comes to a halt, and the voiceover explains, "The Martians had no resistance to bacteria in our atmosphere to which we had long since become immune. Once they had breathed our air, germs which no longer affect us began to kill them. The end came swiftly. All over the world, their machines began to stop, and fall. After all that men could do had failed, the Martians were destroyed, and humanity was saved, by the littlest things which God, in his wisdom, had put upon this earth."

Those "littlest things" were the same invisible germs that postwar global health surveillance organizations were dedicated to investigating and containing, and it is unusual that here, they are seen as a beneficent force.

Although contagious disease is an accidental narrative agent in *War of the Worlds*, the control of invasionary forces by institutions of public health is a recurring feature in science fiction films of the 1950s. As noted above, the UN and WHO iconography condensed the utopic and dystopic aspects of global modernization in a single trope. For instance, a newsreel-style voice-over similar to the framing device in *War of the Worlds* also structures *Invisible Invaders* (1959), and at the film's conclusion, after the invaders have been conquered, the heroes are celebrated at a special UN meeting. Over documentary exterior shots of UN headquarters and interior shots of the assembly hall, intercut with studio shots of the film's cast, the reportorial voiceover intones the moral of the story: "Earth had been on the brink of disaster. But out of the holocaust of war, in which a dictatorship of the universe had been defeated, a lesson had been learned. The nations of the world *could* work and fight together, side by side, in a common cause." Ironically though, before the triumphant globalization sequence takes place (earth's inhabitants band together to defeat the enemy from outer space), a distinct but equally iconographic sequence occurs. In a montage of documentary newsreel footage, international scenarios of destruction—exploding buildings, bridges, dams, radio towers, and automobiles—are attributed to the wrath of the invading aliens, as the transportation and communication networks which provide the essential infrastructure for globalization break down.

Thus, before the regulatory agents of globalization can rescue humanity from alien colonization, the foundations of their power have already been undermined. Through this convention, documentary stock footage invests the sequence with its realism, while the actual threat of global invasion can only be expressed through special effects or otherwise artificial representations of the invading aliens. Similarly, before the WHO saves the day in *The Eternal Fight* (1948) or *The Silent Invader* (a 1957 public health film discussed in chapter 4), the film demonstrates the impossibility of halting the spread of invisible contagions across national boundaries, precisely because of their rapid movement through modern transportation technologies.

In postwar public health and science fiction films, contagion metastasizes from local infection to global catastrophe; once the first town is colonized, the alien or viral invasion spreads like an epidemic disease across the entire country and planet. The telephone, telegraph, highway, and airport provide the sole sources of salvation, but at the critical narrative moment the technology fails, the network is already controlled. This narrative crisis is perhaps epitomized by the moment in *Invasion of the Body Snatchers* (1956) when the central protagonists realize that the "pods" already have possession of the telephone lines and that their only hope is "to make it to the highway." And therein lies the deep contradiction of the audiovisual discourse of world health: it denies the possibility of visually representing and thereby containing the invisible contagions that circle the globe, but simultaneously embraces the fluidity of commerce that is attained through such celebrated border-crossing features of postwar globalization as jet airplane travel, television, and satellite communications.

"A STRANGE NEUROSIS, EVIDENTLY CONTAGIOUS"

As in the films discussed above, the preoccupation with scientific realism and the boundaries of visibility pervades *Invasion of the Body Snatchers*. This film, too, is narrated by voiceover, but unlike the others, its voiceover lacks the authoritative qualities of newsreel-style narration. Instead, *Invasion* is structured as a flashback narrated by the character of Dr. Miles Bennell, who is introduced as a hysterical, paranoid madman in the opening scenes of the film. Under police restraint in a hospital emergency room, Bennell is interrogated by a doctor from the state mental institution, and the story he recounts forms the plot of the film. Because the "reality" of alien invasion has not yet been confirmed, this opening sequence establishes the character of Bennell as an unreliable narrator. As the hospital scene dissolves, flashing back to the previous Thursday, when the suspicious events began to occur, the authority of his point of view is already undermined. Thus, from the very beginning of the film, a tension exists between the narration and the visual representation of the events that the voiceover describes. This disjunction is underscored by Bennell's own criticism of his perceptive capacities: "At first glance, everything looked the same. It wasn't. Something evil had taken possession of the town."

The problem of misinterpreted visual signs pervades the narration of *Invasion of the Body Snatchers*. Just as postwar public health films are preoccupied with visually identifying invisible signs of contagion, the narrator of *Invasion* is retrospectively preoccupied with his own failure to identify the (seemingly obvious) signs of alien invasion. This failure is particularly striking given the character's profession; as a medical doctor, Bennell is supposed to have expert training in the visual detection of invisible signs of infection. The anxiety produced by Bennell's inadequacy is repeatedly expressed through voiceover admissions of observational failures: "The boy's panic should have told me that it was more than school that he was afraid of. And that littered, closed-up vegetable stand should have told me something, too." The gap between image and reality drives the plot of the film; as the doctor sees patient after patient claiming that family members have been replaced by impostors, the conventionalized faith in the authority of the medical gaze continues to dissolve.[19] The central problem of the film — "there is no difference you can actually see . . . but there's something missing" — thus undermines the traditional boundaries between observer and observed, afflicting both alike.

The elusive element that is "missing" from the impostors is revealed when a partially formed "body snatcher" is discovered on the pool table of another character's (Jack Belacheck's) house. The body appears to be incomplete — it is structurally whole, but has "no details, no character, no lines." In an attempt to fit the mysterious figure into a legible system of signification, Dr. Bennell takes its fingerprints (figures 54 and 55). This technique for obtaining and classifying bodily information collapses the surveillance systems of medicine and law, and the body's refusal of the system, its failure to register identifying marks (it has no fingerprints), abruptly establishes the incomprehensible horror that is beginning to unfold. While this film has often been interpreted as a critique of conformity, the impossibility of categorizing the "body snatcher" through socially conventionalized techniques of bodily investigation suggests that the film also operates as an endorsement of the very institutions of corporeal surveillance that produce this denigrated conformity in the first place.[20] In other words, the film's dependence on normative social structures (represented by the doctors and police of the opening and closing sequences) would suggest that it is actually deviance, not conformity, that is suspect in this film. But whether *Invasion of the Body Snatchers* ultimately celebrates deviance or conformity, it remains in either case deeply suspicious of any disjunction between appearance and reality. Thus, the doctor's inability to link the internal essence of the body with its visible surface is

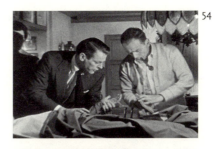

Invasion of the Body Snatchers (1956)

the precise source of the threat posed by the invaders. That is, the body's lack of concrete distinguishing characteristics, the impossibility of differentiating an impostor from a "real" person, demands resolution through an intensified practice of bodily examination. And indeed, when Bennell calls upon a fellow doctor for assistance, that doctor insists (in standard conspiracy film form) that he has to see the body with his own eyes to believe it.

The specific process of bodily invasion is demonstrated when the "pod" at Jack Belacheck's house develops a laceration on its palm in the exact place where the "real" Jack had cut his own hand. This indexical sign of bodily possession functions as a distinguishing mark that defines the boundary between the authentic and the artificial, even as it highlights the instability of that boundary. As an inanimate object, without the indexical body wound, the pod is categorizable (if not comprehensible) as an artificial simulation of the real Jack, but once the concrete stigmata of bodily penetration is conferred upon the invader, the pod simultaneously becomes completely legible *and* makes incomprehensible all systems of signification. The world health demand that bodily surfaces be made legible in order to prevent the global spread of contagious disease is paralleled by the demand, in this and other alien invasion films, that the invisible invaders be detected to prevent them from colonizing the entire planet.[21] But when the indices of individual identity are convincingly simulated by the alien invaders, the demand becomes impossible to fulfill.

When the protagonists of *Invasion of the Body Snatchers* have uncovered the alien conspiracy to replace all of the "real" humans with artificial alien beings that only appear to be human, they devise a plan to halt the invasion: they will search every building in town and examine the bodies of all men, women, and children. Hoping that "whatever is taking place is confined to Santa Mira," Bennell gets on the telephone and asks the operator for the FBI office in Los Angeles. The character's worst fear—"If they've taken over the telephone lines, we're dead!"—is confirmed by the operator's claim that all of the phone lines in Los Angeles and Sacramento are busy or dead. This revelation dramatically intensifies the sense that a global conspiracy is closing in on the film's only remaining humans; the modern communication technologies provide a vital network of bodies, information, and commerce, but they also provide the opportunity for the conspiracy to spread rapidly across the world. Thus, the central contradiction of the discourse of globalization is invoked at this pivotal narrative moment, as the telephone lines that could have sent warnings and prevented the infectious spread of alien invasion are instead used as a system of surveillance: the telephone operator repeatedly rings Bennell's home and office to monitor the resistors' movements. Moreover, one of the most horrifying moments of the film occurs when the sole remaining humans witness the local citizens gathering in the town square, early on a Saturday morning, to receive and distribute truckloads of "body snatcher" seed pods to their family and friends in neighboring towns. The systematic distribution of the invasionary force through transportation technologies parallels the monopolization of the communications networks; as Bennell exclaims, "First our town, then all the towns around us. It's a malignant disease spreading through the whole country!"

Metaphors of disease are frequently employed in interpretations of alien invasion as Communist allegory. For instance, Nora Sayre links the themes of infiltration and conformity in *Invasion of the Body Snatchers* to the brainwashing and mind control that was associated with the experience of prisoners of war in Korea. But she also notes that "Communism was often compared to fatal illness" in this period, citing a campaign speech made by Adlai

Stevenson in 1952, in which he claimed that Communism was "a disease which may have killed more people in this world than cancer, tuberculosis, and heart disease combined."[22] And note the slippages from chronic disease to contagion to Communist allegory in this account of Cold War cinema by David Seed:

> The operative metaphor in these films of invasion as disease was already politicized by the 1950s. "Cancer" had become a catch-all term "for any kind of insidious and dreadful corruption" and J. Edgar Hoover had railed against the Communist "infection" spreading into American life. *Body Snatchers* attempts to straddle mental and physical illness when the town psychologist diagnoses a "strange neurosis, evidently contagious, an epidemic mass hysteria." Jack Finney has denied that his novel had anything to do with the Cold War; but the pods can be read as a metaphor of perceptions of Communism as emotionless regimentation, or subservience in a production and distribution system.[23]

Furthering the rhetorical linkage of invasion and disease, Michael Rogin associates postwar consumer culture with the dialectic of visibility and invisibility in his discussion of Cold War films, arguing that the cinema of this period simultaneously "distinguished subversives from countersubversives" and highlighted the "emergence of a mass society that seemed to homogenize all difference and make subversives difficult to spot."[24] The centrality of surveillance mechanisms—specifically, disease and national or bodily border surveillance—to the discourse of world health is matched by the perpetual failure of those mechanisms to detect the invisible signs of difference that make contagion (or subversion) "difficult to spot."

As Raymond Williams has influentially argued, the expansion of electronic technologies of representation throughout the public and private spheres in the postwar period resulted in a breakdown of the boundaries between those spheres; Williams called this phenomenon "mobile privatization."[25] Two key elements of this historical shift were the mobility offered by affordably mass-produced automobiles (in which members of the "affluent society" could drive to their new tract homes in the suburbs), and the privacy offered by the newly accessible television (which allowed virtual contact with the world from the seclusion of one's own home).[26] The intersection of transportation and communications technologies that enabled "mobile privatization" to occur was also central to the development of the discourse of world health, with its emphasis on the technological successes and failures of globalization. And it is precisely through these technologies that the conspiracies of alien invasion films are carried out.

The flow of contagion through global transportation and communications technologies might productively be linked to the concept of televisual "flow" developed by Williams and taken up by numerous theorists in the field of television studies. The widely noted anxieties about the contaminating effects of television viewing, seen as both emasculating the male viewer and contributing to the overall deterioration (understood as feminization) of culture, bear obvious similarities to the discourse of film spectatorship as contagion in the 1930s. In both cases, what is taken to be the passive posture of spectatorship makes the viewer especially vulnerable to psychological and physiological infection by the images on the screen. This scenario operates through the obverse of the world health logic that "representation equals inoculation"; here, representation of aesthetically or morally impure images equals bodily contamination, and the only kinds of bodies that are seen as weak enough to be vulnerable to such contamination are—whether male or female—feminized. Because the bodies that are subject to this form of possession in postwar science fiction films are predominantly male, this logic repeatedly produces "homosexualized" male protagonists.

The sexual implications of these technologies of globalization were extensively thematized in public health and science fiction cinema of the 1950s, but they are largely absent from the standard interpretations of the genre. This absence is especially surprising given the prominence of both heterosexuality and homosexuality in popular discourse in the years following the publication of the Kinsey reports (1948 and 1953), with their scandalous allegations of widespread sexual "perversion" among average American adults.[27] In a notable exception, Michael Rogin has argued that science fiction films were particularly popular during the Cold War period because these films addressed anxieties that underlay the more explicit worries about Communism—namely, anxieties about the influence of mass culture itself. However, Rogin ultimately links invasion to gender and heterosexual difference, not to homosexual contagion, which, as I will explain below, is central to the evolving discourse of world health. As Rogin argues, "*Body Snatchers*, like *Manchurian Candidate*, united deceit with bodily invasion and located both in female influence."[28] These anxieties play out in the films discussed above through their contradictory attitudes toward globalization. On the one hand, the films celebrate global transportation and communication technologies for their ability to eliminate geographical distance and political difference; but on the other hand, the films blame the very same technologies for failing at crucial narrative moments and thereby enabling the enslavement of the human race by alien invaders.

The global flow of information and commerce that characterizes mobile privatization represents both salvation and doom in *Invasion of the Body Snatchers*. When Bennell finally does make it to the highway, a steady rush of cars passes him by, without heeding his warnings or stopping to help. And when he finally does hitch a ride, it is in the back of a truck full of seed pods, heading out of Santa Mira. Returning to the emergency room scene that opened the film, we find the psychiatrist about to have Bennell committed, when an ambulance driver brings in a crash victim, casually mentioning that, "We had to dig him out from under the most peculiar things I ever saw. . . . great big seed pods." At this evidence that Bennell's story was true, the doctor grabs a policeman, demanding, "Get on your radio and sound an All Points Alarm! Block all highways and stop all traffic and call in every law enforcement agency in the state!" But our knowledge that the communications technologies have already been infiltrated by the body snatchers undermines any sense of narrative resolution that this proof of Bennell's sanity might have delivered. Instead, the film ends with the ominous implication that it may already be too late: the global networks may already be under alien control.

GLOBALIZATION AND ALIEN INVASION

Because these films are fundamentally concerned with the question of how to discern visible evidence of the interior corporeal truth of an individual, the dialectic of visibility and invisibility is as central to postwar science fiction cinema as it is to the public health films discussed in chapters 1 and 2. While public health films ask whether a subject is healthy or diseased, science fiction films want to know whether a subject is human or alien. As we have seen, the question of whether a foreign (immigrant) body would be treated as human or alien has long been at the core of discourses of immigration and disease. The determination of a body's citizenship status (and consequent subjectivization or dehumanization) depended upon a public health officer's visual surveillance of that body's hidden corporeal truth, its internal "essence." In early-twentieth-century discourses of immigration and contagion, and in mid-twentieth-century discourses of alien invasion and contagion, the interior of the body was a privileged object of anxiety—an invisible space that was nonetheless constantly under surveillance. It is this preoccupation with imaging the body's interior that links the public health project of investigating the body with science fiction's obsessive representation of that body's invasion by alien beings.

As noted above, a recurring characteristic of alien invasion films is the failure of transportation and communication technologies at pivotal narrative moments. The globalization of these networks, especially in the postwar era, produces a crucial contradiction for the discourse of world health: transportation and communication networks both enable and prevent the rapid spread of contagious disease across national borders.[29] In science fiction films, the spread of invasion or contagion is initially local but ultimately global; once the first town is completely colonized, the invasion will spread across the entire country. The protagonist consistently turns to the telephone (or telegraph) and the highway (or airport) as the sole means of escape, only to find that the networks have already fallen to the conspiracy. This failure encapsulates the contradiction of globalization, on one hand enabling limitless hybridity, variation, and heterogeneity of culture, while on the other hand producing a transnational corporate conspiracy leading to capitalist monopoly and cultural homogeneity based on consumerism without borders.

In a variation on the theme of globalization as contagion, it is a pair of telephone repairmen in *It Came From Outer Space* (1953) who are first possessed by the alien invaders. The possession takes place just after an amateur astronomer (John) and his girlfriend (Ellen) question the repairmen about whether they had witnessed any unusual occurrences that day. The previous night, a romantic interlude between John and Ellen had been interrupted by what seemed to be a giant meteor crashing into the desert. The couple enlists a helicopter pilot to bring them to the site, and there, John descends into the crater and discovers what appears to be "some kind of a ship," with a creature moving inside of it. At this crucial moment of visual surveillance, a rock slide occurs, covering up the ship and almost killing John. The occlusion of the evidence sets the dialectic of visibility and invisibility in motion; when the hero reaches safe ground, neither his friend nor his girlfriend believes what he saw, and he cannot produce any visible proof. Thus begins the conventional antagonism in alien invasion narratives: between the hero who has seen or can see the truth and the rest of the ignorant and suspicious townspeople, who think he is crazy.[30]

Having been ridiculed by the local press, police, and even fellow scientists, John and Ellen depart the scene of the landing and drive along the desert highway. An abrupt and seemingly unmotivated cut from a lateral tracking shot to a high-angle aerial tracking shot from behind the car, accompanied by alien theme music (the omnipresent science fiction theremin), appears to mark a shift in perspective to the alien point of view (figure 56). However, a different alien point of view had been marked, in an earlier scene (when John was investigating the "meteor"), by a blurry, gelatinous framing device that aligned the camera with the monocular visual perspective of the alien. Translucent concentric circles distorted the edges of the visual frame while the object of the alien's gaze looked directly into the camera, terrified at what he saw looking at him (figure 57).[31] This aerial tracking shot along the highway, which is aurally coded as the alien point of view, lacks the distinctive visual marking of the previous subjective camerawork and yet seems to represent the alien perspective. The next cut presents the car passengers' perspective, as a strange creature appears before them on the highway. The car screeches to a halt, John and Ellen get out, unsure of what they saw, and find nothing. But another subjective alien point-of-view shot, complete with rippling edges, visually signals that the alien is watching them, although they cannot see it (figure 58).

The next day, when the main characters come upon the telephone repairmen working on a line along the desert highway, one of the repairmen explains that he's been hearing a strange and unidentifiable sound over the telephone lines. The fact that others are hearing things, if not seeing them, confirms John's suspicion that "something unusual" is going on and prompts

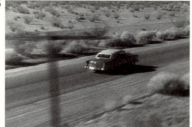

56

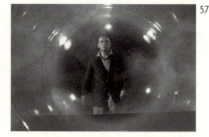

57

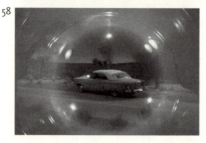

58

It Came From Outer Space (1953)

an investigative drive along the highway in search of clues. As the telephone repairmen scout the opposite direction, the view of their truck suddenly shifts to the same aerial tracking shot that was aurally coded in the earlier scene as an alien point of view, and they, too, come upon a strange creature in the road. When they get out to have a look, the thing swallows them in a smoky cloud.

Throughout the film, the alien point of view is alternately aligned with the monocular shot and the aerial shot, but while the former appears to be unambiguously marked and motivated as the visual perspective of the one-eyed alien, the latter shot seems more likely to be a prototypical b-movie attempt at creating a special effect on a low budget: a standard form of camerawork is made strange through the jarring effect of an unmotivated cut, combined with an otherworldly soundtrack. However, the motivation of the seemingly unmotivated aerial tracking shot has in fact been hinted at throughout the film and is visually explicated in a later sequence, when Ellen is driving through the desert alone, at night. A frontal close-up of Ellen cuts to a low-angle long shot, positioned along the edge of the highway to view the car approaching, and when the car passes, the camera pans right slightly, but instead of continuing to pan right and follow the car, the camera stops on a telephone pole, tilting up to the "T" that supports the wires and pausing on this shot. The next cut returns to the aerial tracking shot and theremin soundtrack, this time unambiguously aligning the alien point of view with the telephone lines.[32] This linkage literalizes the collapse of invasion and technologies of globalization: the international telecommunications network enables the mobile surveillance of the entire planet by extraterrestrial invaders. (Amusingly, though, even the aliens are subject to the failures of globalized transportation and communication in this film. As the conclusion reveals, the aliens landed on earth not to invade but, rather, because their spaceship broke down and needed repairs, and they only took over human bodies to acquire the necessary parts at the local hardware store without arousing suspicion.)

The causal linkage of alien invasion with the breakdown of transportation and communications networks is memorialized in *The Day the Earth Stood Still* (1951), a classic of the genre that explicitly locates the threat of alien invasion in the colonizers' potential monopolization of global networks of information and commerce (resulting in the "stillness" of the film's title). Even in films that locate the threat not in technological power but in the dehumanization that takes place upon alien possession, the breakdown of global networks denotes the all-encompassing scale of the catastrophe. *Invaders from Mars* (1953), *Invasion of the Body Snatchers* (1956), and *I Married a Monster from Outer Space* (1958) all contain pivotal scenes in which telephones and telegraphs fail to connect with the outside world, and roadblocks prevent escape from the site of invasion. But the concept of invasion as anti-globalization is extensively thematized throughout *It Conquered the World* (1956). The central character in this film is not physically possessed by the invading force, but he nonetheless willingly cooperates with it, out of misguided (coded as "perverted") scientific curiosity or what the Payne Fund researchers of the 1930s might have called "emotional possession."[33] The character of Dr. Tom Anderson is established at the film's opening as a visionary or crackpot who warns the government that launching a satellite will menace the safety of the entire world because the earth is under constant alien surveillance, and the launch will be perceived as an act of aggression that will provoke retaliation. Here, a technology meant to facilitate the globalization of communications networks is represented as the direct cause of alien invasion, and indeed the alien travels to earth using the satellite itself as its mode of transportation.

In a montage sequence often repeated in the invasion genre, the alien's arrival in *It Conquered the World* provokes a global collapse of transportation and communications technologies. This conventionalized sequence includes images of clocks, trains, newspaper presses, cars, and industrial equipment all grinding to a halt, images of presumably dead phone and electricity lines, followed by close-ups of fingers tapping apparently unresponsive phone receivers. This abstraction of the local crisis into a worldwide catastrophe links alien invasion with the failures of globalization, but it is strikingly similar to the sequence in *The Eternal Fight* in which the same technologies are represented in a montage of successful prevention of invasion (by contagious disease). But here, instead of offering salvation, these technologies bring doom. When we return from the montage to the local scene, we find that all of the cars, telephones, and radios have failed except for those belonging to Dr. Anderson. With a virtual monopoly over the town's mobility and communications, the alien utilizes his willing servant to organize the distribution of electronic control devices that attach to the backs of their victims' necks and subject them to the will of the alien. Once possessed, the "key control people" in the film (the mayor and chief of police) become zombie-like automatons who round up the local townspeople and force them into reprogramming "camps" in the middle of the desert.

While the alien's control over transportation and communication technologies is crucial to the "conquering" of the film's title, the alien only gains access to the key sources of power through the assistance of the "emotionally possessed" Dr. Tom Anderson. The control of global networks of power is thus vitally linked to human seduction by the alien other. Because of the persistent interlacing of contagion with national and bodily invasion in world health and science fiction cinemas, the process of boundary crossing is frequently conceived as sexualized, often resulting in the simultaneous expression of homosexual panic and desire. The acts of alien possession are often staged through conventionalized imagery of seduction: as illicit encounters in isolated locations such as dark street corners and parks that take place after a night of drinking or marital strife. It might seem unlikely that the more abstract processes of globalization would also be sexualized in these films, but the acts of bodily and national boundary crossing are collapsed, and both are presented as direct effects of the cinematically fetishized technologies of global communication and transportation.

For example, the recently constructed Palomar Observatory telescope figures prominently in science fiction films of the 1950s, as a space-age technology of surveillance more powerful than any previously available on earth.[34] In *Invaders from Mars*, the telescope is a key site of countersurveillance; at a pivotal narrative moment, the observatory functions as a staging ground for organizing resistance to the alien invaders. The telescope's powerful capacity for visual surveillance offers safety by returning the alien gaze, but it also offers a different kind of visual pleasure. In the midst of a suspenseful conspiracy narrative, driven by the desire to visually discover the invisible aliens, the representation of the telescope abruptly freezes the narrative for an extended display of the spectacular object, accompanied by a romantic orchestral soundtrack. The camera fixes upon the telescope's dome, rotating in slow motion in a sequence that perfectly—but oddly—illustrates Laura Mulvey's description of the classical Hollywood conventions for fetishizing the female body. Mulvey's critique of the alignment of narrative movement with "masculine" activity and spectacle with "feminine" passivity might seem ill-suited to an analysis of technology as spectacle—after all, the dominant cultural coding of science and technology is gendered masculine, and the genre of science fiction tends to affirm that coding.[35] And yet, the visual representation of the Palomar telescope is only one example of the extent to which technology nonetheless occupies the place of the "feminine" within the "masculine" domain of science fiction cinema.

While it is ostensibly the alien and not the representational apparatus that is being investigated in these films, the generic requirement of alien invisibility shifts the focus of the scientist's gaze back onto the technology itself. This shift is produced as a consequence of the aggressive (though seemingly pleasurable) bodily invasion enacted by the aliens, which undermines their status as passive, "feminized" objects of spectacle. It is precisely this reversal of traditional subject-object gender coding that places the male scientists in the precarious position of becoming themselves the objects of the alien gaze. To dispel this threat of "feminization," the focus of the cinematic gaze is shifted, and its fetishizing effects are redirected back onto the technologies of globalization. Through this slippage, the few and already marginalized female characters in these films are displaced altogether by the alien technologies of invasion and possession, and a homoerotic regime of visuality is set firmly in place.

BODILY POSSESSION AND HOMOSEXUAL CONTAGION

In science fiction films, as in many public health films, boundary crossing is specifically understood as a threatening form of bodily penetration. When the alien-invaded body, which is usually male, becomes the fetishized object of the cinematic gaze, "penetration panic" becomes "homosexual panic."[36] Consequently, alien invasion is often heavily coded as homosexual contagion, and by collapsing alien and sexual difference (understood in this context as deviance) these films enact the Foucauldian claim that sexuality is linked to the hidden "truth" of the subject. The narrative search to visualize the invisible alien thus becomes a search to reveal the contaminating difference hidden within the body of the seemingly "normal" subject. And central to this endeavor is the protagonist's capacity to transcend the limits of visual perception.

In many of the alien invasion films of this period, the effects of possession register imperceptibly within the victim's body, but usually a residual trace of the invasion is left on the body's surface. This trace functions as an erotic sign marking the boundary between alien and human, a visible signifier denoting the border between the real and the imaginary. In *Invaders from Mars* and *It Conquered the World*, a mark on the back of the victim's neck denotes the point of entry, but in *It Came from Outer Space*, *Invasion of the Body Snatchers*, and *I Married a Monster from Outer Space*, the trace is not left on the body of the possessed, but rather, it is represented through the doubling of that body. For a significant portion of these films, two corporeal forms coexist: one animated by the agent of invasion, the other lifeless, in suspended animation (literally and figuratively). When the aliens in *It Came from Outer Space* and *I Married a Monster* take over a human form, they leave the "original" empty but unharmed: throughout the films, an extra set of bodies populates the outskirts of town. At the climactic moment of narrative resolution, when these "extra" bodies are discovered, a doubling effect that lingered offscreen throughout the film is finally made visible onscreen.

The trope of body doubling has two key implications for my analysis. The production of an extra set of bodies as a by-product of alien invasion can be seen as a displacement of the compulsion to visualize the invisible. The failure to secure an indexical image of the invisible interior truth of the body (is it carrying a contagious disease? is it an alien?) results, in public health films, in a proliferation of "artificial" images of the imagined contagious disease. Here, the same failure results in a proliferation of bodies—not only does every possessed human have an extra (alien) body inside of it, but there is also a hollow replicant of that same body lingering offscreen.[37] This doubling also has important implications concerning the sexual politics of these films. The metaphorical "double life" of the closeted homosexual resonates in this context not only because the dialectic of visibility and invisibility can help to explain what Eve Kosofsky Sedgwick has called the "epistemology of the closet," but also because, in the alien invasion genre, homosociality becomes homosexuality precisely when the male characters' bodily boundaries are "penetrated" by the alien invaders.[38]

As with all of the various forms (and residues) of possession, the uncanny effect that simultaneously alerts perceptive observers and throws their sanity into question is the effect of familiar townspeople not being themselves, and yet not being visibly different from themselves. The central protagonist of every alien invasion film is distinguished by his or her unique ability to see, to observe visual signs that are invisible to the other characters in the film. This perceptive observer will detect the invisible signifiers of alien possession, and the search for visible signs of this hidden internal essence will provide the film's narrative drive. The dynamic between internal and external signs of difference is crucial to the surveillance of contagion that drives the discourse of world health, not only as articulated in scenarios of immigrant medical inspection at national borders, but also as articulated through the dialectic of visibility and invisibility in postwar public health films. The same compulsion to visualize invisible contagions that drives promoters of world health to continually attempt (and fail) to map the spread of disease also drives the alien invasion genre, in a displaced form. All of these films are preoccupied by a search for "the real," and in both the public health and science fiction films, the moment of revelation turns not on the indexical capturing of a profilmic "truth," but rather, on special effects. In public health films of this period, animated signs of disease "prove" that germs really exist (while simultaneously registering the impossibility of locating an indexical sign of contagion), while in the alien invasion films, special effects (including animation) reveal the visible difference that was invisibly present all along, when the alien invader departs the human body and appears in its true form.

As noted in chapter 2, Michel Foucault's linkage of systems of bodily surveillance with the "deployment of sexuality" reveals the process by which the hidden "truth" of a subject has come to define that subject's position within scientific, medical, and juridical systems of knowledge and power: "Thus sex gradually became an object of great suspicion; the general and disquieting meaning that pervades our conduct and our existence, in spite of ourselves; the point of weakness where evil portents reach through to us; the fragment of darkness that we each carry within us: a general signification, a universal secret, an omnipresent cause, a fear that never ends."[39] Just as, in *Hemolytic Streptococcus Control*, the implied threat of homosexuality was linked to the global spread of invisible contagions, in science fiction films it is linked to the global spread of alien invasion. The contagious conspiracy to colonize earth is facilitated by alien control over both "emotionally possessed" men and global transportation and communications technologies. The trope of alien possession invokes the dialectic of visibility and invisibility; as the conspiracy spreads and suspicion mounts, the surface of every body is scanned for visible signs of difference, for evidence of the alien hidden inside the apparently human body. Because alien possession leaves minimal traces of the act of bodily invasion, the manifestations of difference are often located at the level of interpretation, and specifically, the interpretation of signs with ambiguous meanings. Thus enter the themes of paranoia and conspiracy: is her husband sneaking off into the woods with other men at night, or is she just a crazy or possessive or bored housewife? Given the setting of the alien invasions within the heteronormative domesticity of small-town America, the external signs of internal difference are often conceived in sexual terms—the sign of alien possession is a male character's alienation from his wife and implicit sexual affinity for other "possessed" men.

In her influential account of the "epistemology of the closet," Eve Kosofsky Sedgwick locates the distinction between sexual difference and other forms of "invisible" difference in the contagiousness uniquely attributed to homosexuality: "When gay people in a homophobic society come out . . . it is with the consciousness of a potential for serious injury that is likely to go in both directions. The pathogenic secret itself, even, can circulate contagiously *as* a secret: a mother says that her adult child's coming out of the closet with her has plunged her, in turn, into the closet in her conservative community."[40] Sedgwick emphasizes that while the revelation of a previously unknown Jewish identity (for example) will not provoke an anxiety that the person to whom the revelation is made will be implicated in the other's "Jewishness," the revelation of homosexuality does carry the implication that all who are exposed to this secret will become infected themselves.[41] From this perspective, postwar alien invasion films provide an excellent example of how the "epistemology of the closet" illuminates the linkage of the dialectic of visibility and invisibility with the national and physical boundary anxiety that pervades and defines the discourse of world health.

Returning to the sexual undercurrents of *It Conquered the World* alluded to above, the invading alien in this film establishes contact with earth before it arrives, using the character of Dr. Tom Anderson as its intermediary. The "mad scientist" has constructed a machine that tunes in radio signals from Venus, and he claims (to his disbelieving wife and colleagues) that he can discern and comprehend a "voice" within the high-pitched sound waves transmitted over his speaker. Soon, Tom begins to converse with the alien, listening attentively to its language of electronic tones, and telling it, "It's true, I am your only friend. Nobody else even knows you exist." The alien interruption of heterosexual romance that pervades the genre (as when the spaceship crash interrupts a marriage proposal in *It Came from Outer Space*) is epitomized by a scene in this film when Tom's worried wife, Claire, tries to pry her husband away from the communication device, alluringly clad in a silky negligee. She asks Tom to come to bed, but he responds (attaching gender to the alien being), "He's here, darling. He drew the satellite to his world, to Venus, and now he's back, within an hour. He's inside that circling laboratory just waiting to come down to us. To save us." Tom's wife treats his claims of intergalactic interchange as a sign of illness, pleading, "Please come to bed. You'll feel better in the morning." Claire's incessant fidgeting with her wedding ring underscores the specifically sexual nature of the threat posed by the alien; while Tom reluctantly tells it that he's signing off and will reopen contact after sunrise, he refuses to accompany his wife to bed, telling her that he'll "stay by the set tonight."[42]

The alien's origin on Venus, the planet named for the Greek goddess of love, instead of the conventional Mars (the war planet, with its generically typical "little green men"), hints further at the sexual quality of the threat posed by Tom's passionate desire for knowledge of this "exotic" other. Tom's intimate designation of the object of his obsession as "him" reveals the set of displacements that occur in this film: when the homosociality of Tom's affinity for the alien male links up with the dialectic of visibility and invisibility that defines the boundary between human and alien, Tom's scientific curiosity, his desire to know the alien, is transposed from homosocial to homosexual desire. Moreover, despite Tom's unique exemption from bodily penetration by the alien, his "emotional possession" is still treated as a sign of infection; when Tom ecstatically receives a transmission from the alien, telling him it survived the crash landing of the satellite, Claire responds, "Tom, you're a sick man." Tom tries to call after his wife as she storms out of the house, disgusted, but he is interrupted by the alien in a triangulation that occurs throughout the film.

The sexual displacements of this film come into stark relief during the one scene in *It Conquered the World* that (almost) directly addresses them. While Tom's desire for the alien has been construed as scientific curiosity and Claire's jealousy has been represented as concern over her husband's sanity, the "real" meaning of the alien invasion comes out in the sequence when Tom explains to Claire the process of alien possession. Telling his wife that the alien "benefactor" sends out "control birds" that attach radio-like transmitters to people's necks, subjecting them to the alien's will, Tom represents this act of penetration and conversion as an epiphanic moment of bodily possession. When Tom celebrates the elimination of emotion that comes with alien possession, but tells Claire that he'll "need" her even when no emotion exists, an unexpected outburst follows that jarringly breaks with the tone of the film. Claire cries out, "I don't see why you should [need me]. . . . For a few dollars you can hire a woman who will fit all your fetishes. She'll match your requirements perfectly. And if you ever get tired of her, you can always run down to the employment agency for another!" This abrupt shift in discursive registers suggests that we've suddenly cut from a science fiction film to a "sexploitation" film. But the oddness of the exchange is significant: the scene seems strikingly out of place, despite the profusion of sexual innuendo throughout the film, precisely because the desire that is driving the narrative is *not* a heterosexual desire, as is conventionally the case in classical Hollywood cinema. While Claire's outburst is predicated on her perception that Tom's passion for the alien "other" constitutes a heterosexual form of marital infidelity (thus the suggestion that he simply get a prostitute to fulfill his "needs"), Tom's mode of discourse with the alien suggests a qualitatively different form of desire—a desire that his wife and friends simply cannot understand.

As Sedgwick has explained, it is precisely the *invisibility* of homosexuality, in contrast to the visibility of most other forms of difference, that structures the unique forms of anxiety attached to sexuality: "Vibrantly resonant as the image of the closet is for many modern oppressions, it is indicative for homophobia in a way it cannot be for other oppressions. Racism, for instance, is based on a stigma that is visible in all but exceptional cases . . . so are the oppressions based on gender, age, size, physical handicap."[43] Thus, even on a narratively implicit or unconscious level, the trope of sexual deviance is invoked in this set of films as the most widely comprehensible, "commonsense" mode of representing a hidden, internal pathology. The slippage from homosociality to homosexuality that is produced as a result of alien bodily invasion structures the cause-effect chains in *It Conquered the World* and *I Married a Monster from Outer Space* (see below). But even when "the closet" is not a central narrative element, (homo)sexualized alien possession drives numerous other films of the genre. The structure of the closet is integral to the narrative structure of conspiracy, which fuels not only science fiction invasion films, but also public health films that represent the impossibility of containing the spread of invisible contagions. But even as a secondary theme, the visible/invisible epistemology of the closet permeates the science fiction invasion genre. For instance, although the aliens in *Invaders from Mars* possess men and women alike (and even children), the scene in which the primary causal event of the film takes place is heavily infused with "closeted" implications.

The morning after the child protagonist (David) in *Invaders from Mars* has sighted what he believes to be a flying saucer, his father George goes missing. On the previous night, George had told his wife (Mary) that he was going to investigate the boy's story because "the work at the plant is secret, and we have orders to report anything, and there have been rumors." His wife wants to know where her husband is going, and why he has to investigate in the middle of the night, but he won't tell her anything more. The next morning, after the worried wife has summoned the police to search for her husband in the sandpit beyond the house, George suddenly reappears, still in his nightclothes, bedraggled, missing a slipper, and with a zombielike stare. The implication that George has spent the night engaged in inappropriate activities, away from his socially sanctioned marital bed, is underscored by the secretive defensiveness with which he greets all questions concerning his whereabouts and the conspiratorial tone with which he greets the policemen when they return. Moreover, David notices a red, x-shaped scar on the back of his father's neck—a sign of the bodily penetration that occurred while he was out in the middle of the night.[44] When the policemen return from their search, they agree that if George is "feeling ok," they won't report the incident. David notices their scars, too—a sign not only that they are participating in a homosocial conspiracy, but also that, if everything is indeed "ok," then they all must have willingly submitted to this form of unsanctioned bodily invasion.

When Mary offers coffee to the policemen, her husband abruptly cuts her off, with a chastising, "Don't be silly, Mary. These gentlemen have some important work to do." Mary's suspicions are raised when the policeman replies, with a meaningful look, that George, too, has important work to do, and as soon as the officers leave the house, she demands to know what's going on: "What were those men talking about? It's as if you were in some kind of a plot together!" George refuses to explain, instead dragging Mary out to the pit to convert her to alien control. At this point, the homosociality of the plot is replaced by a more generalized conspiracy. While the male homosocial plot does not structure the entire narrative of *Invaders from Mars*, its prominent position in the opening sequence of the film serves to establish the importance of male bodily invasion to the paranoia that drives the rest of the film.

The linkage of bodily possession with contagion is explicitly thematized later in the film, when a local doctor rescues the young protagonist, David, from his alien-possessed parents. As the parents attempt to remove their son from the police station, where he has gone for help, the doctor intervenes, announcing, "I'm Dr. Blake from the City Health Department and your son is in my care." When David's mother counters, "What has he been telling you? He's been reading those trashy science fiction magazines—he's completely out of control!" Dr. Blake replies, "It may interest you to know, Mrs. Mac-Clean, that your son is running a high temperature. His heart action is unnaturally fast. It's too soon to tell, but there's every symptom of polio, and I'm having him removed to the isolation ward of the general hospital." Despite the statistical decrease in incidence of contagious disease, and the increase in cases of chronic disease in the postwar period, contagious diseases—especially polio—figured prominently in the American social imaginary of the 1950s.[45] The use of contagious disease as a *ruse* in this film is telling; the polio excuse works precisely because it is based on the dialectic of visibility and invisibility. The doctor claims to have detected—based on her own institutionally authorized observational capacities—the presence of an invisible contagion within David, and this hidden, internal "truth" cannot be conclusively affirmed or denied without the assistance of technologies of representation that are beyond the scope of the naked eye.

"THERE'S NO WAY OF TELLING WHETHER ANY GIVEN MAN IN TOWN IS A MONSTER OR NOT!"

The homosocial/sexual conspiracy resulting from the displacement of the woman by the "male" alien is particularly central to I Married a Monster from Outer Space, for reasons perhaps made obvious by the quintessential B-movie title. This film has been analyzed in terms of its gender and sexual politics, and indeed there is much to be said about the genre as a whole centering on the disruption of suburban heterosexual coupledom, particularly in the context of postwar struggles over the status of women in the public sphere.[46] While my analysis will share this focus on questions of gender and sexuality, it will do so from a somewhat different perspective. I am particularly interested in the articulation of sexuality to discourses of globalization and world health, with their fears about the penetration and dissolution of national and bodily boundaries. As I have argued above, these fears are expressed through a contradictory celebration and anxiety over the globalization of transportation and communications technologies. The continual crossing of national boundaries by these technologies threatens to undermine geopolitical barriers against invisible contagions, thus leaving national and bodily borders vulnerable to a form of invasion that is symptomatically articulated as homosexual panic.

I Married a Monster from Outer Space is, as the title suggests, the story of a young couple that is about to be married when the husband is possessed by an alien. The unsuspecting wife marries him anyway, and when she soon begins to notice strange differences in her husband, she tearfully attributes them to the bleak reality of married life. From the opening scene of the film, heterosexual coupling is represented as a burdensome task that men must submit to and pretend to enjoy, while secretly bemoaning their fate in the company of other men. The true desire of all men, to be without women and with other men, is thus revealed to be the open secret of this film (and of the alien invasion genre as a whole).

As the central male characters gather for a bachelor party the night before Bill and Marge's wedding, the main topic of conversation is the oppressiveness of the institution of marriage. When Bill leaves the group at the end of the night, a companion remarks, "Aw, he's such a nice guy—it's a shame it has to happen to him." The tone of gender antagonism pervades the film (all of the women want to get married and have babies; all of the men want to avoid it like the plague), but an interpretation of *I Married a Monster* simply as an allegory of postwar gender struggle would miss the equally central emphasis on vision and visuality that drives this and many other films in the alien invasion genre. The preoccupation with exploring the boundaries between the seen and the unseen links this film to the public health films that compulsively pursue visible signs of invisible internal differences, especially in the film's construction of alien invasion as an undetectable "homosexualizing" contagion.

The problem of vision is linked to sexuality when, after the wedding, the couple almost collides with another car as they drive to the honeymoon hotel. Bill had not turned on the car's headlights, and when Marge asks how he could see in the dark, Bill responds defensively that he "forgot" to turn on the lights, avoiding the question of how he could see in the first place. Enhanced visual perception on the part of the alien is matched by diminished percep-

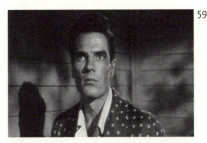

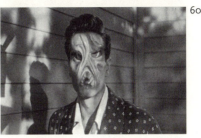

*I Married a Monster from
Outer Space* (1958)

tion on the part of the human (Marge), who is trying to identify the invisible difference that marks Bill as "not Bill." The audience is given privileged access to the hidden internal truth, however, during an awkward scene in the honeymoon suite, where neither the virginal Marge nor the alien Bill knows how to proceed toward consummating their vows. As Marge waits in bed, Bill lingers on the balcony, drawn to the thunder and lightning storm that reveals the alien lurking beneath Bill's human surface: when the lightning flashes, a special effect superimposes a sinewy, vein-streaked alien visage (figures 59 and 60). For a brief moment, the boundary between the seen and the unseen is dissolved through an exchange of the indexical for the artificial, but when Marge calls Bill inside, his human face returns, as does the film's anxious failure to visualize the invisible.

The contrast between visible surfaces and invisible interiors is emphasized throughout the film; the impossibility of representing the invisible is both affirmed and denied at several key moments through the intervention of imaging technologies. From the honeymoon scene, the film jumps ahead one year, to a desperate and disillusioned Marge writing a letter to her mother, describing her inability to interpret the change in Bill: "It has been a horrible year. I'm frightened and bewildered—maybe it's me, but, oh mama,

Bill isn't the man I fell in love with—he's almost a stranger." The impossibility of visually confirming this invisible otherness is underscored when Marge crumples the letter, seemingly admitting the futility of her search for the "real" Bill. The tension between surface and depth is emphasized through a cut from this scenario of secrecy and denial to a close-up shot of an abdominal X-ray—an image that reveals the hidden interior of Marge, not Bill. In her search for visible evidence of the difference that lays within Bill's body, Marge looks inside of her own body instead, playing out Sedgwick's theory of homosexual contagion while remarking, "That doesn't look like me at all!" The doctor's response articulates the crucial role that bodily boundaries play in constituting the desire to visualize the invisible: "If you were turned inside out, that's the way you'd look."

In the discourse of world health, contagion only spreads when it is invisible; the compulsion to visualize invisible contagions is driven by the aim of preventing the penetration of national and bodily boundaries by an invisible invader—if the invader were made visible, its movement could be stopped. In a fruitless effort to reveal the invisible agent that has infected her marriage, Marge submits her own body to the imaging technology of the X-ray, but no clues are found. When the dialogue reveals that Marge's visit to the doctor has been prompted by worry over a "sexual dysfunction"—the lack of conception after a full year of marriage—the (homo)sexual element of the dialectic of visibility and invisibility comes to the fore.[47] The irony here is that the X-ray is used to confirm the absence of contamination within Marge's body; by visually representing her invisible interior, Marge's body is made safe from contagion—her bodily boundaries are secured. But it is precisely this absence of a sign of contagion that confirms Marge's suspicion that a contaminating difference is hidden within Bill; the lack of a sign of Bill's sexual potency (in the form of a fetus within Marge's womb) confirms the "perverted" sexual quality of the invisible invader that has made Bill "not Bill."

When Marge haltingly attempts to convey the doctor's suggestion that Bill, too, should expose his hidden interior truth to the technologically enhanced medical gaze, she explains her discomfort by saying that, "I never know how you're going to react to anything anymore. If it weren't so silly I'd say you were Bill's twin brother from some other place." Here, the recurring trope of doubled bodies symptomatically links the alien invasion genre with the epistemology of the closet. At the suggestion that his (alien) closet be opened (through exposure to the X-ray), so that his sexuality may be scrutinized for reproductive inadequacies, Bill becomes hysterically enraged. But in the midst of the argument about the couple's failed sexual relationship, the doorbell rings, and Bill's old drinking buddy Sam is at the door, claiming that he needs to talk business with Bill. This sequence not only repeats the alien interruption of heterosexual romance identified in *It Came from Outer Space*, *It Conquered the World*, and *Invasion of the Body Snatchers*, it also performs all of the (homo)sexual implications of the contagion anxiety mapped out in *Hemolytic Streptococcus Control* in chapter 2. In the exchange between Bill and Sam, Sam occupies the position of the knowing subject; not only does he know his own "truth," he knows Bill's secret as well. Sam knows that both men are really aliens, and he conveys this knowledge through suggestively sexualized double entendres that Bill refuses to comprehend.[48] Through a sequence that is heavily coded as a seduction, Sam persuades Bill to admit their shared secret, so that he may enjoy his position within the male homosocial alien conspiracy. After Sam's suggestive remarks and knowing glances fail to secure the suspicious and evasive Bill's complicity, Sam becomes more overtly flirtatious and conspiratorial, directly invoking the logic of the closet by asking, "Make many mistakes at first?" When Bill still doesn't "come out," Sam shifts the conversation to bodily invasion itself, complaining about how poorly designed and awkward human bodies are, and telling Bill, "They've improved the methane reservoirs in these bodies. You're due to report to the ship tonight." But Bill continues to act confused, asking Sam how much he's had to drink, so Sam "comes out" to Bill, revealing the alien visage hidden beneath his human surface. At last, Bill admits their shared secret, the two men smile at each other, move closer together, and Bill whispers to Sam, "Well, congratulations."

In Adam Knee's analysis, the dialectic of visibility and invisibility in this film could point to a homosexual conspiracy, but it could just as easily point to other forms of "difference":

The formation of this alien male conspiracy is such that it readily invites allegorical readings in relation to a number of subcultural groups perceived as alien in fifties America. The alien subculture could readily be read, for example, as a gay one, given its emphasis on clandestine all-male meetings and its shared secret knowledge, as well as Bill's inability to consummate his marriage, his quietness and sensitivity, and his evident preference for male companionship, often in the dark. The secretive, plotting nature of the group, in conjunction with its evidently collective consciousness (these aliens, like so many others, communicate telepathically), clearly aligns it with the popular perception of Communists as well.[49]

While Knee's interpretation productively links this film with important social and political events of the 1950s, the fluidity that he attributes to his allegorical interpretation ("otherness" could be sexual, political, or, as later argued, racial) elides the centrality of discourses of visuality and contagion to the alien invasion genre, and, indeed, to postwar American culture as a whole. The crucial interconnection of invisibility and contagion in the figure of the closet points to the centrality of impermeable sexual boundaries to narratives of invasion. Indeed, immediately following the "coming out" scene, Bill sneaks out of the house in the middle of the night, and Marge follows him into the woods (a jealous wife trailing a husband she suspects of having an affair). Marge finally does witness the visible evidence of the difference that she had detected in Bill, when the alien emerges from his body to return to the ship. The inanimate, hollow shell that is left behind topples at Marge's touch, and then, supine in the dirt, it doesn't even twitch when a cockroach scampers across its face. Witnessing this horrifying revelation, Marge screams and runs back into town, trying to find someone who will believe her story, but everyone tells her she's hysterical, insane.

This visual revelation of Bill's hidden corporeal truth provokes a desperate attempt to employ the networks of communication and transportation to halt the spread of the conspiracy. But the generically conventionalized technological failure that results suggests the impossibility of preventing invisible invasions from sweeping the planet. As in *Invasion of the Body Snatchers*, Marge attempts to call Washington, D.C., but the operator tells her that all of the lines are busy. Realizing that the telephone network is part of the conspiracy, Marge hangs up and goes to the telegraph office to send a message to the FBI. But as she departs, Marge sees the Western Union clerk tear up her message instead of sending it. Giving up on the communications networks, Marge takes to the highway, but the road out of town is closed. As she reaches the blockade, a police car pulls up in front of her, and the officers explain robotically that the road ahead is washed out, despite her panicked, desperate objection that it hadn't been raining.

Eventually, Marge gives up and returns home, where she confronts Bill. He explains to her that the alien men of his planet have come to earth to mate with human women. In Knee's interpretation, this scene articulates the widespread racism of postwar America by locating the horror of alien invasion in the white woman's womb; the suggestion of sex between two different species (human and alien) is a displacement of the "horror" of miscegenation, sex between two races—"black" and "white." As Knee argues, expanding on his hypothesis that the conspiracy could be read as gay or Communist:

> Perhaps the most significant metaphorical association of the group is with racial others in white America. Bill eventually explains to Marge that the aliens' goal is the propagation of their race through breeding with human women, and when she asks what kind of children they will be, he responds, "Our kind." The exchange articulates both white fears of the rape of white women by non-white men, and the perception that the progeny of any white-non-white coupling will be non-white.[50]

Knee bases his interpretation on the historical context in which the film was produced; the widely reported—and televised—developments in the civil rights struggle brought racial "otherness" to the fore of white American social consciousness in the late 1950s.[51] And indeed, the sexualized imagery of alien invasion does suggest a linkage to contemporaneous debates about racial "mixing." However, the film's preoccupation with boundary crossing is paralleled by an antagonism toward heterosexual "intercourse" of any kind, from the very opening scenes. While the narrative is structured by the threat that the alien invaders pose to heterosexual coupling and reproduction, the severity of that threat is undermined by the fact that, before the aliens even arrive, the human men are already bemoaning their fates as husbands. Moreover, the central "metaphor" of the film is most pointedly displayed when Marge's horror is contrasted with the alien-men's pleasure as the film's secret is revealed; the displacement of women throughout the film suggests that if this film allegorizes any form of difference, it is primarily a sexual form of difference. But in either case, the slippage from homosociality to homosexuality in this film is not an unambiguous "reflection" of the historical period. Rather, this displacement is a crucial mode of representing anxieties about border crossing—anxieties that were permeating popular and scientific cultures in this period. In many cases, these anxieties were directly concerned with racial border crossing; indeed, sexual reproduction cannot be understood in isolation from racial reproduction. Thus, we see the same slippage occurring in public health films, sometimes emphasizing sexual pathologies, other times emphasizing racial difference, but always driven by fears about the spread of contagion across national and bodily borders.

Despite the film's consistent displacement of heterosexuality, the conclusion of *I Married a Monster from Outer Space* reverts to the ideology of classical Hollywood style. When Marge returns to the doctor, seeking assistance in her fight against the aliens, he reluctantly believes her story, but is concerned that "there's no way of telling whether any given man in town is a monster or not." However, recalling that the first sign of Bill's "otherness" was his failure to produce a child with Marge, the solution to finding visible signs of the invisible alien becomes clear: the doctor realizes that heterosexual impotence is the sign of a man's alien possession, and the scene ends with the doctor marching off through a door marked "maternity ward waiting room," to gather a mob of "real men" to attack the aliens' ship.

CONCLUSION

The shared concern with scientific realism and the boundaries of visibility in public health and science fiction films is articulated through a representational system that I have described in earlier chapters as a dialectic of indexicality and artificiality. The oscillation between documentary footage and animation in public health films is paralleled by science fiction cinema's oscillation between stock footage and special effects. In both sets of films, the process of globalization is represented through imagery of transnational communication and transportation technologies, whose border-crossing qualities situate them in a contradictory discursive position: Globalization is represented as both cause and cure of the spread of contagious disease across national and bodily borders. Or, in science fiction cinema, globalization is represented as both enabling and preventing alien colonization of the planet. The global invasion is paralleled by a local invasion, articulated at the level of the body; the representation of alien possession draws on the same anxieties about national and bodily boundary crossing that pervade public health films.

The thematics of invasion, contagion, and conspiracy that pervade science fiction films of the 1950s—*The Day the Earth Stood Still*, *The War of the Worlds*, *Invaders from Mars*, *It Came from Outer Space*, *Them!*, *Invasion of the Body Snatchers*, *It Conquered the World*, *I Married a Monster from Outer Space*, and *Invisible Invaders*—have been widely understood as representations of American fears of Communist infiltration. In this interpretation (which is often reiterated in popular as well as academic analyses of the period), invisibility is linked to the duplicity of Communist spies, who might pass undetected into the sanctified realm of the suburban nuclear family, and from there, spread their infectious ideology. But as I have argued throughout this chapter, the preoccupation with national and bodily boundaries in postwar science fiction cinema exceeds the explanatory power of the "Communist allegory" interpretation. While the linkage of invisibility with the duplicity of Communist spies suggests that the dialectic of visibility and invisibility pervaded political as well as world health discourses in this period, the prevalence of disease and contagion imagery within the language of anti-Communism suggests that these discourses were inextricably intertwined, not hierarchically ranked.[52]

Moreover, the rapidly expanding realm of postwar consumer culture, particularly mass-mediated audiovisual culture, is also rhetorically linked with the trope of contagion through the technologies of globalization that facilitate both mobile privatization and the threat of transnational conspiracies. The sense that invisible global networks are undermining the security of geopolitical borders is articulated through alien invasions of national and bodily boundaries, and the specific mode of representing penetration invokes the logic of homosexual contagion. As we have seen, the public health mode of representing invisible contagion through a dialectic of indexicality and artificiality is expressed, in science fiction cinema, through a dialectic of stock (documentary) footage and special effects. In both cases, the hidden interior of the body is a privileged object of investigation, and the generically pervasive penetration panic (whether by viruses or aliens) is combated through a proliferation of attempts to visually assert bodily boundaries.

CHAPTER 4

Conspiracy and Cartography:
MAPPING GLOBALIZATION THROUGH EPIDEMIOLOGY

You must be able to see with your mental eye the septic ferments, as distinctly
as we see flies or other insects with the corporeal eye. If you can really see
them in this distinct way with your intellectual eye, you can be
properly on your guard against them.

Hospital Sepsis (1959)

INVISIBLE INVADERS

In the 1959 science fiction film *Invisible Invaders*, an "invisible" race of aliens
threatens to conquer the earth in retaliation for human efforts to explore
outer space. In this film, as in many alien invasion films of the 1950s, the
status of vision and visuality are centrally thematized; the aliens are not actually invisible, but neither are they wholly visible, and the search to determine the boundary between the seen and the unseen provides the central
narrative drive of the film. While few such Hollywood problems reach narrative resolution through "real" science, the degree of overlapping concerns
among postwar medical, scientific, and popular cultures is nonetheless quite
striking. These diverse fields are linked in their preoccupation with visuality,
and, indeed, the "invisibility" attributed to the postwar invaders is belied by
the omnipresent representations of unsanctioned national and bodily border
crossings in this period. Rather than creeping undetected across geopolitical
and subjective boundaries, the imagined invaders announced their presence
everywhere, across a wide range of audiovisual modes of representation and,
crucially, through the discourse of world health.

In this discourse, bodily invasion is collapsed with geopolitical invasion,
and both are treated as processes of contagion. As discussed in chapter 3,
postwar science fiction films represent the process of bodily invasion as part
of an alien conspiracy to conquer the world. The transportation and com-

munication technologies that enable the spread of globalization also facilitate the spread of alien colonization, and thus the very features that define postwar American prosperity and hegemony are ominously revealed to be inescapable global networks of surveillance and social control. By promoting international border surveillance as the solution to the global flow of (contaminated) bodies, information, and commerce that characterize postwar globalization, the discourse of world health espouses an impossible task: to visually represent the invisible paths of transnational contagion. But the same technologies of globalization invoked by the science fiction films also occupy a contradictory status in public health films, as they simultaneously facilitate the spread of invisible contagions and enable the use of surveillance imaging that is meant to halt their spread. In public health and science fiction films, the alien and viral invasion spreads (literally and figuratively) like a highly contagious disease, across the entire planet.

Significantly, in both fictional and nonfictional accounts of global contagion, the spread of infection is neither unpredictable nor accidental. In their endless striving to visually represent the invisible paths of contagion, postwar public health films not only utilize "artificial" means of producing "indexical" representations of contagion, they also invest the invisible contaminant with agency and intentions. While Hollywood films like *Invisible Invaders* represent the spread of alien invasion by intercutting stock footage and special effects, public health films like *The Silent Invader* (1957) narrate the spread of invisible contagions by intercutting documentary footage and animated epidemiological maps. And by plotting the movement of invisible contaminants across the planet, these films invest contagion with malevolent intent; far from randomly flowing from one available vector to another, invisible contaminants are construed as an invasionary force, seeking entry to the United States through any means necessary. Thus, when the ostensibly scientific process of epidemiological mapping is practiced upon seemingly conscious viruses, the pursuit of public health takes the form of a conspiracy narrative. And Hollywood conspiracy films, in turn, borrow the imagery of contagion that drives the pursuit of world health.

In the films I discuss below, conspiracy provides a narrative structure for articulating disease to nationality by explaining processes of invasion and global contagion in epidemiological terms. This chapter begins with a brief historical account of the role of two key representational technologies—cartography and cinema—in the practice of disease surveillance, especially after World War Two. Linking the ambiguous indexicality of cartography with the crisis of signification that characterizes conspiracy theory, I will examine the function of the epidemiological map in public health films, arguing that the failure to secure an indexical image of contagion drives the discourse of world health toward increasingly paranoid narrative forms.

A BRIEF HISTORY OF GLOBAL HEALTH SURVEILLANCE

The desire to monitor, regulate, and visually represent the spread of contagious disease in the public sphere has driven the pursuit of public health since its earliest days. The history of global health surveillance dates to at least 1851, when the first International Sanitary Conference took place in Paris for the purpose of coordinating maritime quarantine requirements intended to prevent the spread of plague, yellow fever, and cholera in Europe.[1] The perceived need for such an organization was linked to the development of transportation and communication technologies, whose reduction of temporal (and perceived spatial) distances led to the increased potential for the rapid spread of communicable diseases.[2] Around the same time, the scientific organization of information into statistics was gaining popularity as a method of classifying and controlling the natural world. Population density maps of social and cultural phenomena had been developed in the 1830s, mapping such demographic characteristics as poverty, crime, sanitation, and disease, and it was through the innovative application of cartographic principles to public health in 1855 that the vector of contagion was first discovered in an outbreak of cholera in London.[3] By plotting individual cases on a city map, a cluster of infections was revealed to center around a single contaminated water pump. This discovery led sanitarians to remove the handle from the offending pump, thus effectively terminating the outbreak. Significantly, this advance in the spatial mapping of disease did not lead to the discovery of the bacterial etiology of cholera but, rather, to the displacement of contagion onto an object that was not actually the true cause of disease.[4]

By visualizing the previously invisible spread of contagion, the epidemiological map assisted in delineating the boundaries between sanitary and unsanitary zones of the public sphere, and this development was part of a broader impulse toward taxonomy and statistical mapping in the nineteenth century. As Allan Sekula has demonstrated, the archival impulse of this period was exemplified by the work of Sir Francis Galton, a statistician who developed the techniques of photographic criminological phrenology while simultaneously applying these principles to his cartographic work at the Royal Geographical Society of London.[5] The centrality of cartography to the early practice of public health reveals the desire to map and thus to regulate the flow of bodies in the public sphere that has driven health surveillance throughout its history.[6] In chapter 1, I noted the intersecting institutional histories of public health and cinema; here, we can see the importance of cartography—another ambiguously indexical form of representation—to the public health regime of visuality.

The regulation of entry into the United States also became increasingly systematized starting in the mid–nineteenth century. By the 1850s, all states with busy ports of arrival had instituted systematic inspection procedures, including quarantine of the sick. Public health policy was focused primarily on preventing the introduction of contagious diseases into the United States from abroad; even diseases that were endemic to North America were treated as alien threats.[7] After several meetings of the International Sanitary Conference, a permanent committee, the Office International d'Hygiène Publique was established in 1907. The OIHP coexisted with two other international health organizations—the Pan American Sanitary Organization (founded in 1902) and the Health Organization of the League of Nations (created in 1923, in the aftermath of World War One)—until the World Health Organization (WHO), created by the United Nations in 1948, unified and absorbed the activities of all three organizations.[8]

The Communicable Disease Center (now the Centers for Disease Control and Prevention, known as the CDC), based in Atlanta, Georgia, also developed out of World War Two. In the postwar period, a heightened public concern over the position of the United States in relation to an imaginary global map of world health was answered by the transformation of the United States Public Health Service (USPHS) agency, Malaria Control in War Areas (MCWA), into the permanent institution of the CDC in 1946.[9] In the late 1940s and early 1950s, CDC transitioned from working on specialized projects in war areas to addressing a broader range of contagious diseases threatening peacetime national security. As with the return of troops after the Spanish American War and World War One, the global travels of servicemen during World War Two raised concerns about the invasion of United States soil by "exotic," invisible diseases carried within the bodies of returning soldiers. The enormous expansion of air travel in this period exacerbated these fears; consequently, training programs in the control of communicable diseases also expanded during the postwar period.[10] Among other projects, the CDC developed a training program for public health field workers that acquired global significance as it attracted an international array of students. The program made extensive use of audiovisual materials in order to "eas[e] the language problems"[11] attendant upon opening the program to participants from around the world. These films served a variety of ideological and logistical purposes, including instructing field workers in methods of epidemiological surveillance, popularizing hygiene techniques among U.S. schoolchildren, mobilizing mass campaigns for smallpox vaccination and eradication in West Africa, and instructing male soldiers and civilians in methods of preventing the spread of venereal diseases.[12]

By establishing clinical sites and field offices in previously colonized countries, the CDC and the WHO began incorporating local populations into transnational systems of knowledge, charting the intersections of contagion, physical bodies, and geographical locations onto a global map of hygienic modernization. The films produced by these organizations thus occupy important positions in the worldwide spread of Western ideologies of bodily surveillance and control. In the same period, cartography regained its mid-nineteenth-century prominence, but this time serving (at least some) as an anti-imperialist tool. As Geoff King has noted, "The national atlas was revived as a potent symbol of nationhood after the 1939–45 war when the format was used by a number of newly independent states. The new states were merely turning to their own advantage cartographic techniques that had been used repeatedly by colonial powers to legitimate their territorial claims."[13]

But not all postwar mapping practices served anticolonial aims; the CDC's transnational reach is epitomized by one of its prominent programs, the Epidemiological Intelligence Service (EIS), which was created in 1951 to gather information on diseases around the world and to provide expert assistance to health-related crisis zones and "infectious disease emergencies" anywhere on the planet, upon request.[14] While the project undoubtedly demonstrates a degree of benevolent internationalism, that aspect of the EIS also disguises its strategic importance to Cold War surveillance activities; funding for the service was secured, in part, to ensure U.S. preparedness for the potential development of biological weaponry during the Korean War.[15]

The global scale of the CDC's (and the WHO's) pursuit of public health created an enormous demand for personnel trained in specialized health surveillance techniques, which presented, in turn, the need for a universal language of international communication. The shortage of experts available to respond to the suddenly urgent demands of world health prompted the CDC's further investment in efficient and mass-reproducible technologies of instruction; the transnational dissemination of training in the techniques and ideology of world health could only be accomplished through the use of audiovisual aids.[16] Consequently, the medium of film attained a uniquely privileged status in promoting world health during and after World War Two.[17] Audiovisual materials had also played a crucial role in the CDC's prehistory as MCWA—the organization first employed instructional films in order to rapidly train a huge staff in the techniques for eradication of malaria-bearing mosquitoes during World War Two.[18] After the war, CDC training films were in such high demand that the organization launched its own production studio, as the postwar assistant surgeon general proudly proclaimed in his history of the USPHS: "The most complete and up-to-date equipment available for production of superior films, filmstrips, and slide series has been installed in the audio-visual production services of the center and well-trained technicians in this field have been employed. A film library is maintained which lends training films and filmstrips to health agencies and schools throughout the world."[19]

From this perspective, we can see that the CDC's prestige as a preeminent postwar global health surveillance organization was perhaps defined as much by the center's mastery and distribution of audiovisual technologies of representation as it was by the CDC's "control" of infectious diseases. Furthermore, the CDC's media empire reached both scientific and popular audiences; the USPHS also produced a series of health education motion pictures "for the information and guidance of the general public," during the postwar period.[20] When new headquarters were constructed for the CDC in 1960, an entire building was dedicated to the audiovisual unit, containing two large sound stages, several darkrooms, and a state-of-the-art sound department.[21]

As noted above, medical cartography had been of central importance to the practice of public health since the 1855 cholera outbreak, but like the medium of film, the epidemiological map attained a new prominence after World War Two. While global health surveillance organizations were producing moving images of the transnational flow of contagions in the postwar period, the American Geographical Society was simultaneously working to popularize thematic cartography amongst the general public. To that end, the society published an innovative series of maps between 1950 and 1955 "showing the world distribution of cholera, dengue and yellow fever, leprosy, malaria, plague, polio," and other contagious diseases.[22] Meanwhile, the films produced by postwar institutions of public health were collectively preoccupied with epidemiological cartography to the extent that virtually every cinematic treatment of infectious disease included an animated map of contagion.

By the mid-1960s, the Audiovisual Unit of the CDC was no longer part of the center's Training Branch—it had become a separate unit of the USPHS and was re-named the National Medical Audiovisual Facility (NMAV). In 1967 President Johnson secured an enormous budget for NMAV by selling the program to Congress as the way "to turn otherwise hollow laboratory triumphs into health victories."[23] The perceived need for the USPHS to demonstrate the relevance of its activities to the general public through popularized motion pictures that explain those "otherwise hollow laboratory triumphs" is particularly revealing when considered in relation to contemporaneous events in the mass media. The sharply critical "Vast Wasteland" speech delivered in 1961 by Newton Minow, chairman of the Federal Communications Commission, had prompted the development of a new era in television production, and during this time, "quality" shows and "relevant" programming were meant to replace the mindless drivel that Minow claimed had characterized television programming up to that point.[24] The television networks' widely noted attempts to provide socially and politically conscious programming for a presumably intelligent audience affected other spheres of cultural life as well; President Johnson's efforts to link scientific progress with social progress through the films produced by the NMAV indicate a recognition, on the part of federal policy makers, of the close association between audiovisual modes of entertainment and audiovisual modes of education. This ideological intersection parallels the formal and stylistic intersection of public health and Hollywood modes of representation, not only in the science fiction films discussed in the previous chapter, but also continuing from the 1970s to the present day, in representations of global contagion as global conspiracy.

DOCUMENTING CONTAGION: EPIDEMIOLOGICAL CARTOGRAPHY

In chapter 2, I discussed the ontology of the image of contagion as it oscillates between indexical and artificial modes of representation; here, I will bring that dialectic to bear on a key iconographic feature of the audiovisual discourse of world health: the use of epidemiological cartography to represent the temporal and spatial flow of invisible contaminants. In postwar public health films, the problem of world health is presented through a dialectic of visibility and invisibility, articulated through two generically characteristic representational techniques. First, the spread of infectious disease is conceptualized as a problem of global proportions by linking contagion with transnational communication and transportation technologies, whose assistance in both monitoring and spreading disease is demonstrated on animated epidemiological maps of the world.[25] The mutually reinforcing conditions of universal surveillance and universal contagion produce a model of globalization that absorbs the United States into the seemingly unstoppable flow of infections and, consequently, defines the ideal of "world health" as an untenable contradiction. This stalemate is resolved through the second representational strategy, which works by constructing a visual icon of disease that enables the displacement of contagion onto sources outside of the United States, even while infectious agents continue to move freely across national boundaries. By locating the origins of disease in so-called Third World countries, and intercutting world maps with documentary images of the inhabitants of those nations (as visible evidence of the presence of invisible contaminants), these public health films recuperate the dystopic fatalism of globalization by quarantining diseased bodies within the spatially and temporally distant locales of "premodernity."

On animated maps of the global spread of disease and in documentary footage that codes nonwhite bodies as disease carriers, the actual contaminant (whether bacterium or virus) remains invisible. What is made visible is not an indexical image of invisible contagions but, rather, a socially legible — albeit entirely artificial — collapse of the invisible onto alternate forms of representing disease. The constant oscillation between these two modes of representation produces a form of realism that strives to attain an authoritative indexical status while nonetheless relying heavily on nonindexical modes of representation. Thus, we arrive at a key contradiction in the audiovisual discourse of world health: the aim of global health surveillance is to trace visually the spread of contagious disease, thereby sustaining the imaginary geopolitical map that establishes a spatial and temporal evolutionary gap between the scientifically advanced "modern" world (of the West), and the disease-ridden "premodern" world (the rest of the globe). Such maps reify the literal and figurative relationship between these two worlds as that of scientific investigator and lab specimen. However, the inherent instability of the relationship between observer and observed leaves the practice of surveillance always inadequate to the task of preventing "foreign elements" from entering even the most highly guarded national and bodily borders. Despite (or perhaps, because of) this contradiction, the medium of film is mobilized by health surveillance organizations as a technology of visualization that can capture images of germs that are invisible to the naked eye and then re-present them to a mass audience, training an entire nation of viewers in the techniques of disease surveillance and epidemiological mapping. The instructional power of public health films ostensibly derives from their status as scientific documentations of reality, and yet these films cannot actually capture an unmediated profilmic scenario of contagion without displacing the invisible contagion onto artificially constructed visual images.

The epidemiological map raises special problems for the world health preoccupation with capturing authentic profilmic images of contagion. On one hand, a map is an abstracted representation of reality that only ever exists in mediated form. Whether handmade or computer-generated, a map is always "artificially" constructed, and thus it is impossible to produce a map through processes of photographic realism. That is, one cannot create a map simply by photographing a mass of land; in order to transform the photographic image into a map, it must be manipulated, altered by interpretive markers that integrate the image into a legible system of signification. For this reason, I describe maps as "ambiguously indexical" signs. On the other hand, historically, maps have functioned precisely as indexical representations of reality; their use value in navigating and claiming sovereignty over unmarked territory is demonstrated by the age of exploration and colonization, and the political effects of the presumed objectivity of cartography rapidly follow. Much as Louis Althusser described the interpellative function of ideology, Geoff King has noted that "the national map and the concept of nationalism are inextricably linked," and Denis Wood has described the function of maps as "the ceaseless reproduction of the culture that brings them into being."[26] Thus, historically and semiotically, maps occupy an intermediary, liminal position between indexicality and artificiality; they delineate imaginary boundaries with real material consequences, while simultaneously blurring the boundaries between image and reality.

The figure of the map has also occupied a central position for theorists of poststructuralism and postmodernity.[27] In Jean Baudrillard's oft-cited quotation of Jorge Luis Borges, postmodernity is an epoch in which "the map precedes the territory."[28] In other words, Baudrillard argues that reality has been displaced by simulations of reality in the increasingly image-based culture of the postwar United States. This claim has been reiterated by cultural critics and sociologists alike, as Geoff King has observed:

> Concern about the potency of images as against the reality they were thought to pervert or obscure, rather than accurately to map, became acute during the 1950s and 1960s in the West, particularly in the United States. Some years before the term "postmodern" gained any wide currency the growth of media such as television and advertising seemed to some commentators to result in the swamping of a real that became lost beneath a wave of image, fantasy and illusion.[29]

Under these circumstances, "the map [that] precedes the territory" stands in for the artificiality of all representational forms in postwar culture. However, the ability to "map" reality is seen by some theorists as the only possible escape from the superficial meaninglessness of postmodernity. Here again, the ontological status of the map fluctuates between artificiality and indexicality.

A similar crisis of signification has characterized another representational form that has been closely identified with postmodernity: the narrative of conspiracy. Numerous cultural theorists have noted the thematic prevalence of paranoia and conspiracy in postwar literary, cinematic, and political narratives, and as many have identified some form of epistemological crisis at the root of this culturally dominant mode of representation.[30] For instance, Timothy Melley has noted that conspiracy theory "arises out of radical doubt about how knowledge is produced and about the authority of those who produce it," and he argues that the form has been "a fundamental organizing principle in American film, television, and fiction since World War Two. Numerous postwar narratives concern characters who are nervous about the ways large, and often vague, organizations might be controlling their lives, influencing their actions, or even constructing their desires."[31] Often described as a destabilization of referentiality, the search for "truth" (unmediated reality) that drives the conspiracy narrative is based on the same anxious dialectic of visibility and invisibility that drives the discourse of world health. In Mark Fenster's analysis, "as an interpretive practice, conspiracy theory represents an impossible, almost utopian drive to seize and fetishize individual signs in order to place them within vast interpretive structures that unsuccessfully attempt to stop the signs' unlimited semiosis."[32] The impossibility of securing an indexical relationship between signifier and signified drives the theory of conspiracy, just as the impossibility of visually capturing a profilmic image of contagion drives the epidemiological narrative of world health.

The emblematic figures of conspiracy and cartography are joined in the work of Fredric Jameson, who employs the notion of "cognitive mapping" to argue that conspiracy films represent attempts (albeit failed ones) to figure totality in the impossibly complex web of multinational capital that characterizes postmodernity. By focusing on the representation of global social systems through political conspiracies, Jameson conceives of cognitive mapping as a practice that can make invisible global networks visible. While this dialectic is clearly central to the representation of world health, the distinctions in the map's ontological status in each case have important implications. For Jameson, mapping is a figurative process, whereas for the discourse of world health, mapping is both literal and figurative, and at the center of this ambiguity rests the elusive indexicality of the map of contagious disease. Despite its frequent failures, the discourse of world health is dedicated to the project of epidemiological mapping, and this form of scientific positivism would seem to occupy a state of epistemological certainty, not crisis. Although the map of world health is inherently unstable, this instability does not render the world unmappable but, rather, highlights the perpetual flux of all global inscriptions of power. As Geoff King has argued, the supposed "unmappability" of postmodernity can be reinterpreted through reference to a concrete case in recent political history: "The example of the Middle East offers a salutary reminder to those who champion the supposed arrival of a postmodern 'New World Order' in which national boundaries are said to be blurred by an increasingly global economics and culture. Instead we find a dialectical movement between the dissolution and reassertion of boundaries, the erasure and reinscription of lines on the map."[33]

Cinematically, the ambiguous indexicality of cartography extends beyond geopolitics and narratives of conspiracy to represent the fear of alien and viral penetration of national and bodily boundaries. As noted in earlier chapters, this anxiety pervades public health and Hollywood science fiction films, and it is also a key feature of later conspiracy films that engage the discourse of contagion and world health. But while this fear is diffuse and generically pervasive, the representation of bodily invasion is notably linked to a specifically masculine articulation of anxiety. The "homosexual panic" that ensues at the first hint of cinematic penetration of male physical boundaries itself operates as a form of contagion anxiety, and when this threat is cast as an invisible conspiracy of potentially global scope, the paranoia becomes all-encompassing. Typifying this dynamic is the scenario of fetishistic inoculation phobia that repeatedly occurs, even in the midst of deadly epidemics, whenever a large syringe appears onscreen.[34] For instance, several injection scenes in Panic in the Streets (1950) are constructed as film noir gangster standoffs, in which the masculinity of the needle-wielding public health officer (appropriately played by tough-guy actor Richard Widmark) must dominate that of the penetration-phobic police force and longshore-men, who resist vaccination as if they are rebuffing an unwelcome homo-sexual advance.

Timothy Melley has theorized this particular form of homosexual panic as a conspiracy-based, paranoid view of "social controls as *feminizing* forces, domesticating powers that violate the borders of the autonomous self, pene-trating, inhabiting and controlling it from within."[35] Casting this representa-tional paradigm in historical perspective, Melley compares early American "melodramas of beset manhood" with later narratives of paranoia:

> In the postwar period, this tradition becomes coupled to a narrative of violated identity and agency-in-crisis—a story about the implantation of social controls into previously self-enclosed, integral, atomistic sub-jects. Such stories privilege the male body and heterosexual norms in conceptualizing human agency and subjectivity. While the earlier tradi-tion imagines the mechanism of control to be a constraining [feminine] environment, the postwar narrative imagines it as a bodily violation, an *introjection* of the social order into the self.[36]

Significantly, Melley links his description of paranoid fiction of the postwar period with other critical interpretations of the period, including the widely influential work of Jean Baudrillard.[37] The totalizing view of postmodernity as a simulacral system producing depthless subjectivity construes the im-plicitly masculine subject as vulnerable to the excessive proximity of the increasingly image-based postwar American culture.[38] Such traditionally "feminizing" proximity results in the dissolution of protective boundaries, thus threatening all forms of bodily invasion and contagion. In Melley's view, "What Baudrillard finds so frightening about the total system . . . is not only its control of the social realm, but its penetration and 'emptying out' of the individual."[39] But I would add that the expression of masculinist anxiety re-sulting from the blurring of boundaries between image and "reality" is not unique to the postwar period. In fact, the same concern legitimized the so-cial science examination of women, immigrants, and children in the 1930s—the purportedly vulnerable (feminized) members of the motion picture audi-ence whose spectatorial acumen was feared to be insufficient to distinguish fiction from reality. Moreover, an important feature of the discourse of reform (and resulting censorship) in this period was the linkage of film viewing with infection; the regulation of motion picture content to prevent "moral contagion" was designed to eliminate the "reality" from the fiction. Instead of training vulnerable viewers to identify the boundaries between image and reality (between artificial and indexical), and thus secure an appropriate distance from the representational form, the Production Code simply sanitized the image, with the aim of ensuring that the vulnerable viewers' excessive proximity to the realm of the imaginary would not result in physical or psychological contagion.

In other words, the anxiety that Baudrillard attaches to the advent of postmodernity is far from new; rather, it is only the latest version of a highly gendered form of anxiety about the impact of mass cultural technologies of reproduction on individual subjectivity.[40] The postwar emphasis on vulnerable male bodies has been linked to a broader cultural tendency in this period to see male suffering and consequent emasculation as caused by the increasingly powerful status of women (relative to prewar norms) in both public and private spheres. This perceived shift in dominant gender ideologies is exemplified by such popular written texts as *Generation of Vipers* and *The Man in the Gray Flannel Suit*.[41] But, as with the language of film reform in the 1930s, the critique after World War Two of the "excessive proximity of the image" is infused with imagery of bodily invasion and contagion. The cultural pervasiveness of this imagery suggests that in addition to recognizing the crucial transformations of domestic gender relations and consumer culture taking place during this period, one must consider the broader discourse of globalization, cast in the world health terms of national and bodily invasion. While an anxious relationship to mass culture may have informed postwar identity formation, the particular form of this influence suggests that the representation of bodily boundary crossing has subjective implications extending far beyond a new articulation of an age-old form of technophobia. Just as the rhetoric of Communist paranoia was entwined with the discourse of global contagion in my analysis of science fiction alien invasion films, here we see the paranoid critique of postmodern "depthlessness" or "unmappability" interwoven with the ideology of world health. As my discussion of epidemiological mapping in postwar public health films

will show, the fear of bodily violation by invisible pathogens is dispelled—
at least temporarily—by plotting contagion onto animated maps.

MAPPING CONTAGION IN PUBLIC HEALTH FILMS

Epidemiological maps played a crucial role in depicting the "Air Age" of the
1920s as both enabling worldwide modernization and threatening global
disease outbreaks. The early linkage of modern transportation technologies
with contagion is illustrated by the 1924 film *How Disease Is Spread*, which
pointedly cuts from a train station scene to an animated map tracing the path
of tuberculosis across the continental United States. Significantly, though,
this outbreak is contained within the borders of the national map—in this
film, at this historical moment, contagion and globalization are not yet fused
into a single representational form. In contrast, public health films made
after World War Two, such as *Hemolytic Streptococcus Control* (1945), *The Eternal Fight* (1948), *Prevention of the Introduction of Diseases from Abroad* (1945),
The Fight Against the Communicable Diseases (1950), and *The Silent Invader*
(1957), explicitly and consistently map the spread of disease as a global phenomenon. These films exemplify the ambiguous indexicality of cinematic
cartography and their "crisis of signification" produces a paranoid ambiance
that comes to define the mapping of disease in several later Hollywood contagion and conspiracy films, such as *The Andromeda Strain* (1971), *The Crazies*
(1973), *Outbreak* (1995), and *28 Days Later . . .* (2003), to name only a few.

During World War Two, even home-front films like *Fight Syphilis* (1941)
frame their localized instances of infection as worldwide pandemics; in
doing so, the film highlights a key problem of public health in the global
era: the permeability of local, state, national, and continental boundaries.
By bringing the local and the global into direct conflict, the film raises another key question of public health: how to translate the global perspective
into local disease surveillance and prevention activities. While *Fight Syphilis* represents the spread of contagious disease within national boundaries,
the threat is explicitly cast in global terms through the rhetoric of national
security. The film was produced to train World War Two troops in the prevention of venereal diseases, and the central protagonist is a World War One
veteran who has been "crippled by the enemy in the blood." In this film, the

importance of maintaining impermeable national and bodily boundaries is treated as requisite to preparedness for international conflict. Rather than emphasizing the threats posed to u.s. borders from abroad, *Fight Syphilis* is dedicated to training viewers in visually mapping contagion onto the seeming innocence of small-town America; national defense begins at home.

As the voiceover in *Fight Syphilis* warns, viewers must "know the danger spots of the city—the places where the disease begins." A tracking shot of Main Street in a generic small American town dissolves from a sunny daytime scene to a darkened, nighttime shot of the same locale, cutting in to a close-up of a sign for "Joe's Tavern." Panning left to reveal a pair of legs in stockings and high heels below a set of swinging barroom doors, the camera reveals a room full of men and women dancing. With the apparent aim of training viewers to visually identify the spatial locations where contagion festers, the voiceover warns of "The places that infect the city, and infect its people, the places with the easy pick-ups. Yes, these are the danger spots, the places that breed syphilis. Know the other danger spots—the dark, hidden streets, the places that are whispered about." By arguing that locations, not viruses, are the source of contagion, this film hints at the postwar claim that disease resides in premodern locations outside of the United States. Instead, *Fight Syphilis* suggests that within national borders, the invisible contaminant cannot be detected on the surface of the body but, rather, must be identified by its location in suspicious sectors of the public sphere. Many postwar public health films conceive of contagion as a global threat through images of racially marked bodies, thus training viewers to avoid infection by avoiding contact with racial "others." But in *Fight Syphilis*, the viewer is trained not to detect specific types of bodies but to navigate public space according to an imaginary map of infectious and noninfectious zones.

Thus, when a man strolls from Joe's Tavern into a dark alley, pausing as a woman beckons from her window, the shot dissolves to an animated aerial view of a street intersection, which dissolves to another aerial shot of broader scope, showing a grid of several blocks, then the whole town, continually craning upward as the melodramatic voiceover warns, "These are the danger spots. Here, the disease begins. Yes, here it begins. Here a new chain of infections starts, a chain of infection that will take the lives of children to be born, and bring people to hospitals, to insanity, and to blindness. Here it begins." At this point an animated icon of two male-female couples appears in the center of the shot, and lines of infection spread out from them across the grid map. At the end of each original line of infection, a human figure appears and more lines shoot out, with additional victims at the end of each line, as the voiceover continues to describe the spread of disease from "one infected person carrying infection to many people, and the infection spreading from them to countless others." The web of disease carriers dissolves, replaced by one male figure marked "Infected," with four lines spreading from him to four female figures below. This shot dissolves back to the man in the dark alley. From the animated representation of the map of contagion, Fight Syphilis returns to live action footage demonstrating the proper, effective techniques for avoiding and treating infection. Closing with admonitions about the need for self-protection, the film concludes with an image of a suburban home, the prototypical white nuclear family sitting around the dinner table, saying their prayers. The shot dissolves to an animated exterior of the house, tracking back from there to a new map of the United States, this time dotted with icons of suburban homes instead of disease carriers.[42] These contrasting visions suggest that future success and happiness depend upon the viewer's ability to produce and navigate an imaginary map of the menacing zones of the public sphere. And yet, these maps chart an invisible and all-encompassing flow of contagion, endlessly reproduced across the entire nation. The importance of avoiding entrapment in the web of infection is asserted even as the deceptiveness of the "danger spots" is made evident: a street that is harmless in the light of day may easily become threatening at night, just as a seemingly "nice" girl may in fact be a carrier of infection. It is precisely this representational ambiguity—the impossibility of distinguishing between sincerity and artifice, health and disease—that invests this film with contagion paranoia.

When the representational techniques employed in Fight Syphilis are used in public health films of the postwar era, the explicitly global context of the later films imbues the figure of the epidemiological map with added prominence, scientific authority, and paranoia. The menacing quality of the linkage of globalization and contagion is unambiguous in the opening sequence of Prevention of the Introduction of Diseases from Abroad (1945). A montage of transportation imagery—including an ocean liner, a train, and an airplane—is accompanied by a voiceover announcing that "the introduction of diseases from abroad has paralleled in growth the remarkable development of transportation on the sea, on the land, and in the air. The transportation of disease has been assisted and much facilitated by improved mechanical methods, as has the transportation of persons or property." Later in the film, the threatening potential of the global transportation network is demonstrated through the example of yellow fever in the Southern Hemisphere. From a close-up of a mosquito specimen, mounted on a pin and rotating before the camera, the film cuts to an animated map of Central and South America. The voiceover explains, "Although yellow fever has been banished from our shores since 1905, it still exists in South America and Africa, and recent developments in air travel again make it a menace to the United States. To combat this menace, the yellow fever mosquito must be eliminated from ships and airplanes, and infectious persons must be detected and isolated."

This warning is articulated through the dialectic of visibility and invisibility: the animated map of the contaminated southern locales is intercut with aerial shots of a maritime quarantine hospital in a port area. The visual scope of this extreme long shot, which includes a large mass of land, sea, and air, is crucial to the film's claim that globalization is eradicating the spatial distances that had previously enabled national isolation from foreign infections. And yet, these images could only be captured from the distance achieved with the assistance of aerial transportation. Thus, the very technology that presents the threat of contagion is integral to the representation of that threat. A similar contradiction constructs the medium of film itself as both source and cure for contagion in the "education versus entertainment" debates of the 1930s, and the communications and transportation technologies that enabled postwar globalization to occur were also seen as assisting in the worldwide spread of contagion in the 1950s.

The aerial spread of contagious disease is examined in some detail following the mapping sequence. The propensity of disease-bearing mosquitoes to stow away aboard airplanes (thus traveling thousands of miles further than their own wings could carry them) is combated through disease surveillance techniques designed to keep "this dangerous, ever-threatening disease . . . outside our borders." Documentary footage of an airplane landing and releasing its passengers leads directly into an inspection sequence, in which thermometers are used to attain indexical confirmation of the presence or absence of invisible contagion within the bodies of the new arrivals. The plane's interior is then inspected, vacuumed, and sprayed with insecticide. From this scenario of controlled and systematic national and bodily boundary surveillance, the film cuts to an animated map showing lines connecting China and North America, as the voiceover intones, "The opening of air routes to the Orient has created serious problems in preventing the introduction of diseases, particularly cholera and smallpox, into Hawaii and the United States." Here again, the juxtaposition of effective disease surveillance techniques with a global scenario whose scope exceeds the boundaries of regulation points to the paranoid anxiety that treats processes of globalization as narratives of conspiracy.

As this sequence demonstrates, the discourse of world health is driven by the tension between recognizing the inherent permeability of geopolitical borders and insisting on the possibility of fortifying those boundaries against invasion by invisible contagions. The plotting of this tension onto national and global epidemiological maps is meant to serve as a protective measure; if the flow of disease can be made visible through an indexical representational form, the contagion can be halted before it enters national boundaries. However, the ambiguous indexicality of cartography undermines the potency of the image, resulting in the proliferation of animated world maps in postwar public health films.

In *The Fight Against the Communicable Diseases* (1950), an animated globe rotates onscreen while the voiceover explains that "communicable diseases recognize no boundaries, for they've taken their toll on human life the world over." As the globe stops turning, the camera slowly zooms in on North America, eventually dissolving to a map of the United States as the voiceover explains that disease surveillance (and outbreaks) may be national, regional, or local in scope. Cutting in to a close-up of a title on the map ("Danville," denoting a small Midwestern town), the camera then tracks back out to reveal the location of this disease outbreak on the national map, while the voiceover explains that "an epidemic might start anywhere, and reach into many states." But even this representation of an outbreak in a small town in the center of the country is cast in global terms, through comparison with "the 1918 influenza pandemic, which was first recognized in Boston, and within

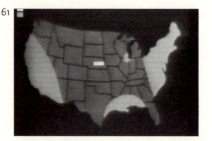

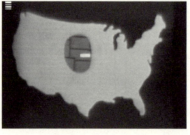

The Fight Against the Communicable
Diseases (1950)

a month, spread throughout the entire country." The threat of universal contagion is dramatically represented here, in an image that has attained iconographic status in the half-century since this film was produced: a map of the
United States fills the screen and as contagion invades the nation's coastal
borders, colored shading spreads westward from the northeast corner, then
eastward from the West Coast, meeting up with waves from the southwest
and the southeast, eventually spreading across and engulfing the entire country (figures 61 and 62). The suggestion that any disease outbreak—even one
that starts in an isolated Midwestern town—could easily result in universal
contagion, casts an anxious pall over the project of global health surveillance.
This anxiety is especially striking in a film that is dedicated to celebrating
the Centers for Disease Control's successful "fight against the communicable
diseases."

In contrast, the triumphant attitude of the World Health Organization
in a segment of the postwar newsreel *A Monthly Review from Europe* (1952)
suggests that the paranoid view of global contagion as conspiracy can be
reversed, in a positivist interpretation of global health surveillance as a conspiracy against contagion. This reversal positions any potential disease carrier in the role of object (victim) of the omnipotent gaze of the global con-

spiracy, but as we will see, this position is constructed as a pleasurable form of security, not a menacing invasion of privacy. In this segment of the newsreel, entitled "World Health," the narrative intersection of conspiracy and cartography in the pursuit of world health is recounted through a case of typhus in the French port of Marseilles. Like *The Eternal Fight* and *The Silent Invader* (discussed below), this film celebrates the global disease surveillance activities of the World Health Organization, simultaneously cautioning against any attempted evasion of the WHO's watchful eye, and applauding the self-regulation of potential disease carriers who internalize the global Panopticon. The film compares the outbreak of an epidemic in Marseilles in 1720 with an outbreak in 1952, promoting the modern techniques of containment that allow efficient and thorough tracking of contagion. "World Health" is a reenactment of the discovery of "sickness, probably contagious," aboard an ocean liner arriving in Marseilles, told through interwoven documentary footage of health inspection procedures and fictional scenarios that create the film's narrative frame. The port health officer responds to the ship's telegraphed warning message by boarding the ship and inspecting its health record. But instead of placing the entire vessel and its occupants under quarantine for two weeks (as premodern methods would dictate), the inspectors subject each passenger to a rigorous modern process of bureaucratic classification. This innovation is designed to elicit the information needed to plot each potential carrier of infection onto a global epidemiological map, thus enabling the inspectors to track past activities, predict future behavior, and prevent further outbreaks.

Documentary footage of the ship's passengers getting their papers stamped by two port officers is explained by a voiceover noting that "for each, a special form is filled in. All vaccinations against contagious diseases are checked from a kind of health identity card, a special form issued by the World Health Organization." At this point, the collection of information in Marseilles is visually incorporated into a global network of surveillance through documentary footage of WHO headquarters in Geneva, where "the United Nations operates its health information center for the world. In the files at Geneva, every known case of contagious disease is recorded and classified. In this way, trends towards even the tiny beginnings of an epidemic can be watched. Then, national officials can decide a control action." The

WHO's capacity for universal surveillance is demonstrated through footage of the organization's detection and classification system, followed by images of two health officers plotting points on a world map, beginning in Africa and tracing lines toward Geneva and across the globe. Over a communications technology montage, the voiceover notes that the information gathered in Geneva is disseminated across the globe by "daily radio broadcasts to all nations."[43]

From the global level of WHO disease surveillance, the film returns to the local case of Marseilles, where a narrative of resistance to the machinery of world health is presented as a pseudodocumentary morality play, demonstrating the necessity of submission to internal and external bodily mapping, in formal scenarios of medical inspection as well as informal leisure activities in the public sphere. Over footage of sailors disembarking from the ship under investigation, the voiceover explains the system of regulation: "Back in Marseilles, all of their data recorded, the passengers of the liner go ashore. Freed, but liable to be recalled at a moment's notice. At the same time, the suspect case goes off to hospital. So far in Marseilles, all is going well." A shot of an ambulance departing from the port cuts to an aerial view of the city, followed by a shot of a taxi pulling up outside a hotel. By intercutting the individual instance of contagion with the broader scope of the city as a whole, this sequence proclaims the mappability of the spread of disease. As a result of the WHO's implied omniscience, the local health inspectors are able to locate the particular in the universal, the infected among the healthy. Having established the impossibility of escaping detection by the ever-vigilant global health police, the film can recount the search for a potentially undetected case of typhus as a lighthearted, even comedic detective story, because the conclusion—that WHO techniques will prevail—has already been established by the documentary footage of the surveillance system at the organization's headquarters.

The event that sets the epidemiological cause-effect chain into motion is the discovery that a passenger from the infected ship has provided the health inspectors with inaccurate information about his planned itinerary. This character, identified only by his first name, arrives at his given address to find that the hotel is full, and he must seek lodging elsewhere. By making a point of preserving the anonymity of the offender ("we'll call him Jean"), the film attempts to establish its own documentary realism, despite the obvious staging of the entire sequence for the camera. Jean's failure accurately to locate himself on the health surveillance map of Marseilles not only provides the first evidence of this character's obvious irresponsibility, but also sets the disease detection machinery in motion. His chance encounter with some friends at a nearby café provides him with a room for the night, and the ensuing celebration only cements his lack of moral fiber—a criminal quality that is underscored by a cut from the scene of Jean's debauchery to a shot of a hospital exterior, where an examination and quarantine sequence takes place: "But then at the hospital, the suspect case becomes a confirmed case. Typhus. Once again there is typhus in Marseilles. But this time, it is under control. Marseilles informs Geneva, Geneva classifies this outbreak, and Geneva informs the world."

The efficiency of the world health surveillance network is demonstrated through another montage of communications technologies. While the fumigation and disinfection machinery moves into gear onscreen, the potential failure of the system is threatened by Jean, the unwittingly resistant subject. Elaborate sequences demonstrating the willing subjection of all passengers to the decontamination procedures are intercut with shots of Jean, strolling the beach and flirting with women, oblivious to the invisible contagion he might be spreading through his implied sexual promiscuity. In order to complete a thorough inspection of all the ship's passengers, a detective is called in to track down the potentially contaminated and contagious Jean.[44] The offender is apprehended, the voiceover explains and "thus, a surprised Jean finds himself in the hands of the police. The charge: his body a possible menace to public health." Jean is reluctantly escorted to the disinfection center, where he "arrives for his spray of DDT." Thus, universal surveillance is shown to effectively prevent the spread of contagion, and while Jean gazes wistfully through the slatted wall of the disinfection center at a woman passing on the sidewalk, the voiceover proclaims victoriously, "As Jean passes into the shower, the now disinfected ship sails once more on a new voyage, on scheduled time. Thus the World Health Organization safeguards and controls, with a minimum delay to trade and transport, and a minimum interference in the lives of people." By promoting self-surveillance as a requisite accommodation to the demands of world health, this film represents epidemiological mapping as a benevolent form of conspiracy. Because no one can escape the watchful eye of the WHO, everyone willingly embraces the ideal of a global health Panopticon, exposing everything so that contagion has nowhere to hide.

The confident affirmation of the effectiveness of global health surveillance in "World Health" is weakly reiterated in *The Silent Invader* (1957). The latter film applauds the work of the USPHS and WHO, even while it represents the United States as vulnerable to attack by an undetectable invader, whose infection of the entire globe may well be unstoppable. Unlike the public health films discussed above, this film deploys racial difference as a mark of contagion, through a representational technique similar to that of *The Eternal Fight* (1948), discussed in chapter 1. While the collapse of contagion and nonwhite bodily surfaces in *The Silent Invader* enables a more visually identifiable mapping of disease, the film's use of epidemiological maps to demonstrate the rapidity with which the invisible invader has circled the globe again raises the specter of global conspiracy. Thus, the film's attempts to assure the audience of U.S. exemption from the impending pandemic come across as anxious, paranoid utterances.

The Silent Invader is a public health film broadcast on television and introduced as "an up-to-the-minute report on Asian influenza." Opening in a conventional newsroom setting, featuring a white male announcer standing behind a desk, in front of a world map, the program immediately launches into a visual montage of "man's battles with nature." This sequence emphasizes the combat mentality suggested by the program's title, as military invasion of national borders is conflated with viral invasion of bodily borders. As in *The Fight Against the Communicable Diseases*, this montage also begins with the influenza pandemic of 1918, noted in the voiceover while documentary footage of World War One troops on the march is displayed onscreen. In the next sequence, various natural disaster scenarios lead into footage apparently shot in Southeast Asia, of a long line of people walking (and being carried) through what appears to be a makeshift hospital or refugee camp, with UNICEF jeeps in the background of the shot. Over this series of images, the voiceover announces, "Unlike the battles of nation against nation, or humanity against the forces of nature, when man has often had an opportunity to prepare himself, the battles against disease throughout the centuries

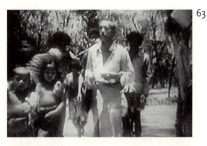

63

The Silent Invader (1957)

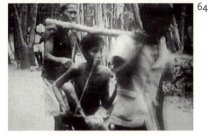

64

have often found man in the unfortunate position of having to combat this enemy only after it had infiltrated his community and infected much of the population."

At precisely the moment when the discursive tone shifts from the agent-less "acts of God" series of natural disasters to the more insidious language of "infection" and "infiltration," the images of nonwhite bodies appear on-screen (figures 63 and 64). Thus, the imagined flow of dark-skinned bodies across u.s. national borders becomes a global flow of infection, and the rhetorical linkage of invasion, infiltration, and infection structures the narration of the spread of contagious disease as a narrative of conspiracy. The linkage of disease and national or racial "otherness" is underscored not only by the documentary convention of the authoritative voiceover, employed here to interpret the visible bodily surfaces of the "Asians" as infectious, but also by the emphasis on global health surveillance as a strategy for delineating the boundaries of modernity according to a geopolitical hygienic hierarchy. Over the display of "diseased" Asian bodies, the voiceover continues:

> You've recently become aware of a pandemic, or a worldwide epidemic, which originated in the Far East and is now known as Asian influenza. Because of the alertness and efficiency of the United States Public Health

Service and the World Health Organization, a detection system, similar to that of the aircraft spotting, has been established throughout the world, and has enabled us to recognize and follow the progress of Asian influenza as it circles the globe.

By suggesting that postwar disease surveillance functions according to the same logic as wartime intelligence, *The Silent Invader* aims to affirm the invulnerability of u.s. national and bodily boundaries.

However, the very title of the program highlights the key paranoia-inducing distinction: airplanes are loud and visible, "Asian" influenza is silent and invisible. Thus, the assertion that geopolitical boundaries can define the distinction between healthy and diseased, modern and "premodern" national identities is both affirmed and denied by this articulation of world health. The very concept of "world health" is founded upon a view of the world as a collection of discrete national bodies, which are nonetheless inextricably interconnected by global transportation and communication networks that prevent any nation from functioning in isolation. This geopolitical web facilitates the spread of disease, even as it promotes the fantasy of universal boundary surveillance and control. The plotting of documentary images of diseased bodies onto epidemiological maps thus performs the crucial function of linking disease with racially marked bodies that occupy geographical locations outside of the national borders of the United States. Through this displacement, bodily invasion becomes national invasion, and the project of world health becomes a world war between modern, "sanitary" countries and disease-ridden, "premodern" societies.

After informing the audience that "health authorities expect an outbreak [of Asian influenza] this fall and winter in the United States," the moderator introduces a professor of public health who acknowledges the impossibility of locating the true origins of the epidemic but nonetheless points out the locations of Hong Kong and Singapore on a world map, indicating that these are the original sources of the disease that now threatens the United States (figure 65). Cutting to documentary footage of streets crowded with pedestrians in those locales, the voiceover narrates the epidemic spread of disease to Formosa, Borneo, Japan, and from the major shipping areas of those places, to widely dispersed locales (figure 66). The first known "invasion" of

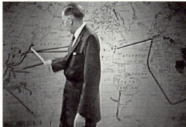
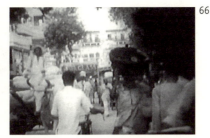

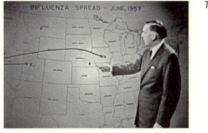

67

The Silent Invader (1957)

the United States was carried on ships from Australia heading toward San Francisco, with the first case entering u.s. national borders "only six weeks after the disease first appeared in China." The rapid progress of contagion is tracked in detail on three consecutive epidemiological maps of "influenza spread" across the entire country in June and July of 1957, providing a visual aid to the narrator's ominous diagnosis of u.s. vulnerability to global contagion (figure 67). By referring to these indexical representations of the spatial and temporal flow of contagion, *The Silent Invader* affirms the mappability of disease, and yet the very facticity of the maps indicates the obvious vulnerability of the United States to universal contamination.

Despite the public health professor's role as the voice of scientific authority, even his narration of the spread of "Asian" influenza is befuddled by the virus's representational instability, its fluctuation between visibility and invisibility. On one hand, the narrator admits that it is impossible accurately to trace the spread of contagion or to impose quarantine because a carrier of the invisible virus may not manifest visible symptoms for days or weeks after infection. On the other hand, the entire program is dedicated not only to identifying the origins of the disease in "underdeveloped" locations outside of the United States, but also to conceptualizing viral contagion as military invasion, thus promoting a racialized form of national defense that chillingly recalls anti-Asian xenophobia during World War Two.[45] In postwar public health films like *The Silent Invader*, the dialectic of visibility and invisibility is expressed through a historically specific form of realism that seeks to produce indexical representations of invisible contagion, but can only produce artificial images of that elusive object. This oscillation between indexicality and artificiality produces an anxious, paranoid mode of representing the flow of contagion, which unambiguously takes on the structure of conspiracy when it is appropriated in later years by Hollywood cinema.

ABSTRACTING INFECTION: FROM WORLD HEALTH TO GLOBAL CONSPIRACY

The representations of contagion in postwar public health films negotiate the problem of invisibility by codifying and visually mapping the infectious zones of the public sphere. Because the spread of contagion involves spatial and temporal mobility, the epidemiological map must account for (at least) two different scenarios of contamination: the geographic infection, wherein bodily presence at a particular location on the map confers contagion, and the demographic infection, wherein contact with a particular type of person results in contamination. While both scenarios are generically codified, their iconography depends upon a discursive slippage that always threatens misinterpretation; whether invisible contagion is visualized through animated maps or through racially and sexually marked bodies, the indexicality of the image of contagion remains unstable at best. Thus, the assurance that these films are meant to provide—as long as you avoid these locations and these types of people, you won't be infected—is easily undermined at the first blurring of representational boundaries. And because the audiovisual imaginary of world health is precisely concerned with the permeability of national and bodily boundaries, these films obsessively represent the dissolution of the very borders that they are attempting to stabilize. The coupling of intense anxiety about the global spread of contagion with representations of (often unsuccessful) attempts to halt the invasion of u.s. borders by invisible contaminants invests these films with a paranoia that structures the narration of contagion as a conspiracy theory. In *Hospital Sepsis* (1959), the possibility of avoiding contagion is completely undermined by the total abstraction of the infectious agent. In this film, there are neither specific types of bodies nor specific locations that are invulnerable to disease. Contagion is everywhere and less visible than ever, and this intensified pervasiveness of infection is only exacerbated by the film's use of sophisticated techniques for visualizing the invisible.

Hospital Sepsis: A Communicable Disease elaborates upon the visual training techniques of the earlier public health films with its emphasis on identifying the spatial and temporal dimensions of contagion. Like many of the films discussed above, this film engages the dialectic of visibility and invisibility through its constant oscillation between documentary footage and animated representation of the spread of disease. *Hospital Sepsis* focuses on the spread of disease within medical facilities, but the film emphasizes the applicability of this particular example to any social scenario by abstracting the training techniques of earlier films that had recommended avoiding specific types of persons or locales (or both), and infinitely extending its scope of contagious scenarios. Not only does the film move away from the bodily marking that identified disease in earlier public health films, but at key moments of tracing the spread of contagion, the film dispenses with human bodies altogether, demonstrating the flow of invisible bacteria without any human carriers at all. And, unlike earlier films that visualized the disembodied flow of contamination with epidemiological maps, this film universalizes contagion through the proposition that where there is air, there is contagion. *Hospital Sepsis* takes as its founding premise the admonition of Joseph Lister, a key figure in the late-nineteenth-century "age of antisepsis," that "you must be able to see with your mental eye the septic ferments, as distinctly as we see flies or other insects with the corporeal eye. If you can really see them in this distinct way with your intellectual eye, you can be properly on your guard against them." From this ideal of internalized disease surveillance, the narrator notes that in the current postwar period of medical and scientific advances, our mental eyes have become lazy, depending too heavily on antibiotics to manage the invisible realm of contagion.

Hospital Sepsis methodically traces the paths of contagion through a case study that effectively manipulates the boundaries between fictional and non-fictional representation. A patient, "Mrs. Allen," enters the hospital with an infected lesion on her arm, and a close-up of the festering sore confirms

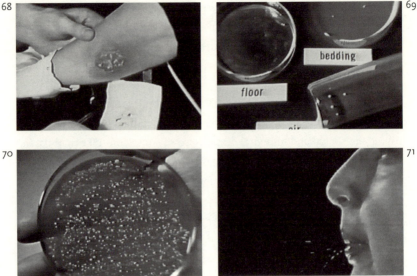

Hospital Sepsis (1959)

the indexical authenticity of the image (figure 68). Before Mrs. Allen settles in, her room is thoroughly disinfected, using techniques that are explained in great detail to the film audience. The success of the cleansing is demonstrated through the first of a series of culture samples, taken from the bedding, floor, and air in the room. These samples confirm their claims through indexical means; when virtually no bacteria appear in the petri dish, we know that the room is clean. Later on, when Mrs. Allen has occupied the previously aseptic room for a day, new samples are taken, and close-ups reveal that they are now filled with bacteria (figures 69 and 70). This technique for visualizing invisible contaminants is distinguished from the use of animation precisely through the indexicality of the discolored sample medium, which proves the existence of germs on the items exposed to the culture. The facticity of the images is further enhanced through the use of a graph to indicate the "increase in bacteria per square centimeter" as Mrs. Allen conducts various activities such as bed making, flushing the toilet, walking down the corridor, and speaking with a nurse (figure 71).

But when the film's discursive register shifts from representing the existence of contagion in isolated locations at specific moments to demonstrat-

Hospital Sepsis (1959)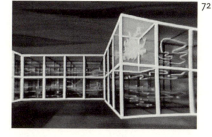

ing the mobility of contagion across space and time, the unambiguous in-dexicality of the contact samples takes on an increased burden of proof. In order to represent the temporal and spatial flow of contagion, the documen-tary images of the scientific experiment are replaced with animation, but the empirically authorized realism of the preceding sequences carries over, in-vesting the animation with the same discursive indexicality as the medium cultures, despite the obvious artificiality of the animated images. As we see an animated, amorphous yellow swath of infection spread through a series of adjacent rooms and ultimately, throughout the entire hospital, a voiceover explains that "if not properly confined, bacteria can travel from the source of infection by dozens of routes. They are carried by feet, hands, clothing, and noses. They circulate by soiled linen and improper ventilating systems. They are spread by blankets, dressings, pails and mops. By any article that enters and leaves the room" (figure 72).

The implication of this sequence and, indeed, of the entire film, is that contagion is omnipresent and therefore unavoidable; viewers must imag-ine the presence of infectious agents in every instance of contact with both animate and inanimate objects, and even then there is no guarantee of ex-emption from infection. The universality of this threat attributes a level of agency to the act of infection that structures the narrative of contagion as a narrative of conspiracy: invisible germs are everywhere laying in wait for their unsuspecting victims.

From this animated explication of the spread of disease, the film cuts back to "documentary" footage of a nurse taking samples from various reser-voirs of bacteria, including a mop pail. The film turns from these indexi-cal images to another animation sequence demonstrating the existence of bacteria, whose presence in the mop pail was only verbally (not visually) af-

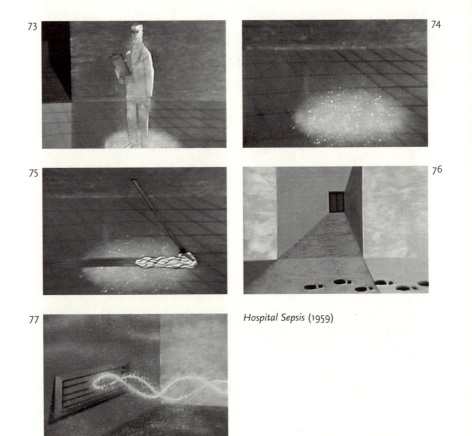

Hospital Sepsis (1959)

firmed in the "documentary" sequence. In the animated sequence, yellow spots trace the spread of bacteria from a person's nose to their hand, to their clothing, and onto the floor. As the yellow infestation trails across the animated figure, the body disappears, leaving a pile of yellow bacteria in its place (figures 73 and 74). From there, the bacteria are picked up on a mop, where overnight they multiply. Despite the film's emphasis on the agency of viewers in preventing the spread of contagion, the bacteria are autonomously mobile throughout the rest of this sequence. The contaminated mop moves without assistance, painting a trail of bacteria throughout the hospital, and when a pair of disembodied feet cross the contaminated hallway, leaving footprints to mark their path, yellow bacterial dust is kicked up into

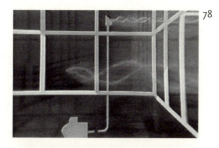

78

Hospital Sepsis (1959)

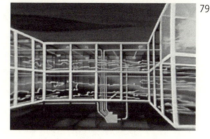

the air vent (figures 75–77). This emphasis on visualizing invisible bacteria by eliminating the bodily vector of contamination reverses the regimes of visuality that have defined the discourse of world health thus far—namely, the dialectic of indexicality and artificiality. Instead, the film fetishizes contagion itself, by simultaneously fetishizing the technologies of representation that allow the image of contagion to take on a visible form.

The consequences of this animated sequence of events are demonstrated through yet another form of indexical imagery; the space of the hallway dissolves into a map of the hospital's ventilation system, tracing the spread of yellow bacteria throughout the entire building (figures 78 and 79). Returning to the "documentary" footage, orderlies are shown mopping and vacuuming Mrs. Allen's room, attempting to prevent the dissemination of particles of contaminated dust into the air ducts. But then a more elaborate animation sequence shows the problems posed by airborne bacteria in stairwells, elevator shafts, and other passageways. The animated images dissolve to an indexical demonstration of the hospital's air currents by showing the movement of smoke (the classic example of the "indexical" sign) through an open door, over a pile of soiled linen, down a hallway, up a stairwell, and into an open nursery door. Despite the seeming success of indexically capturing a profilmic—albeit metaphoric—image of the spread of contagion, at this moment the film returns to animation, systematically demonstrating how the flow of smoke could be blocked at various points of its path.

Two key features mark this film as a turning point in the representation of invisible contagion. First, the use of authentically indexical representational techniques—the petri dish bacterial cultures and the flow of smoke—indicates an intensified effort to close the gap between indexical and artificial modes of representing disease. By closing this gap, the film can more effectively argue the universality of contagion: it can scientifically prove the existence of germs, without resorting to artificial manipulations of the image. And second, the film disavows the notion that contagion can be geographically or demographically isolated. By eliminating the agent of contagion, *Hospital Sepsis* suggests the universality of the threat of infection. Both of these points lead to the film's concluding emphasis on the necessity for subjection to (and internalization of) bodily surveillance. As the voiceover advises, "Each of us must be willing to supervise constantly, and to be supervised. And above all, each of us must be able to see with his mental eye the septic ferments."

As demonstrated in my discussion of alien invasion films in chapter 3, the reliance upon artificially constructed yet scientifically authorized forms of realism in public health films pervades certain genres of postwar Hollywood film as well. I have argued that the dialectic of indexicality and artificiality that defines the cinema of world health is articulated in science fiction films through an oscillation between documentary stock footage and special effects. But in addition, the linkage of alien and viral invasions with technologies of globalization structures both science fiction and public health films as narratives of conspiracy. The emphasis on epidemiological mapping as a strategy for visually tracking the spread of disease, and thus preventing its reproduction, has important repercussions for later representations of conspiracy in popular culture as well. In the resurgence of conspiracy films from the late-1960s through the 1970s, the mapping of invisible contagions is conflated with the mapping of invisible networks of power, and the struggle to make visible the seemingly intangible flow of information and pathology is conducted once again through the epidemiological dialectic of indexicality and artificiality.

CHAPTER 5

Indexical Digital:
REPRESENTING CONTAGION IN THE POSTPHOTOGRAPHIC ERA

And around the world, but especially in the U.S., people sensitized to Ebola's horrors by a spate of books and movies . . . wondered nervously whether the disease would spread out of Africa.

MICHAEL D. LEMONICK, "Return to the Hot Zone"

AIDS is proof that as the 21st century approaches, no virus can be seen as regional and limited—everything from people to plagues circulates the globe.

The Coming Plague (1997)

TECHNOPHILIA AND HOMOPHOBIA

In the public health and science fiction films under discussion here, technologies of health surveillance place the scrutinized body in the traditionally feminized position of visual spectacle. Through their obsessive efforts to identify infectious agents, these films visually dissect the bodies believed to be harboring invisible contaminants. Surprisingly, though, the frequent representation of male bodily invasion does not seem to impact dominant gender norms—that is, until the AIDS epidemic. In fact, it is the female figure, not the male, that critics have traditionally seen as the primary target of cinematic investigation, while male bodily borders are assumed to remain comparatively intact.[1] Historically, this gender dichotomy has been linked to the notion of a uniquely masculine form of unified subjectivity, and consequently has been seen as a source of male privilege and power. As Steve Neale has argued, "While mainstream cinema, in its assumption of a male norm, perspective and look, can constantly take women and the female image as its object of investigation, it has rarely investigated men and the male image in the same kind of way."[2] However, the assumed invulnerability of the male body has been revised in recent years, largely due to the newfound public prominence of imagery of gay male bodies in the context of AIDS. While the "deviance" of this new realm of images might suggest their cultural marginality, the "invisibility" of sexual identity exposes both gay and straight masculinity to this revisionist attitude toward the invulnerability of male bodily boundaries.

Despite the longstanding convention of cinematic objectification of the female body, certain groups of films—such as the science fiction films of the 1950s and the global conspiracy films of the 1970s—suggest unexpected gender reconfigurations. Even prior to the dramatic shift that takes place with AIDS, popular culture's preoccupation with contagion shifts its focus to the universalized male subject of scientific inquiry. Consequently, the feminized specular position is taken over by a male body and contagion becomes linked with homoerotic visual pleasures. By representing contagion through the image of deviant male sexuality, the films I discuss in this chapter—*The Andromeda Strain* (1971), AIDS videos of the 1980s, and *Outbreak* (1995)—conflate the threat of contamination with implied homosexuality, through a trope that often functions as an emblematic form of pathological postwar masculinity.[3] The anxiety generated by the combined pleasures of homoerotic voyeurism and threatened bodily invasion is dispelled through the exhaustive visual dissection of the virus and the use of a "documentary" mode of representation that legitimates the spectacle of bodily penetration by treating it as a requisite component of the discourse of scientific realism. In public health and Hollywood films, it is the act of visual representation that authoritatively establishes the presence of contagion and, through this act of identification, eliminates the potency of the threat of contamination. Given the prestige of the visual in such scenarios, the seemingly unmediated quality of documentary images affords them a privileged position in the representation of contagion, within both fictional and nonfictional narratives. However, the potency of the documentary form depends heavily upon its display of technological mastery over the visual field—a mastery accomplished not only through promotion of its own photographic relation to "the real," but also through a diegetic celebration of the new media that provide technologically enhanced visual access to the invisible contaminants under investigation. Thus, the documentary form can only accomplish its aims by emphasizing the centrality of sophisticated (and highly mediated) representational technologies in capturing its supposedly unmediated visual truth.

As we have seen, postwar public health films are plagued by their failure accurately to capture a profilmic (documentary) image of contagion.[4] It would seem that this problem might be solved by the advent of more sophisticated imaging technologies, and *The Andromeda Strain* attempts to capitalize upon this precise promise. While *Andromeda* exemplifies the articulation of sexuality and contagion in the rhetoric of globalization that begins in earlier science fiction films, it is the film's treatment of "new media" that is most striking. *The Andromeda Strain* fetishizes technologies of visual investigation, dwelling on the dystopic underside of total surveillance by imagining universal contagion as halted only by nuclear annihilation. (In this context, the utopic side of total surveillance is precisely the WHO promise of eliminating disease, preventing contagion, and ensuring good health for all—but here, as in many films of this genre, that benevolent role is occupied by a malevolent government conspiracy to use scientific progress to produce biological weapons.) Most important, though, is the linkage of "new media" with the pleasure of homoerotic visual spectacle—a linkage that provokes the threat of bodily disintegration. In this film, fear of the invisible virus is made manifest as a deadly form of homosexual panic.

The continued desire of the discourse of world health is that the internalization of surveillance techniques will make invisible contagions visible. Paradoxically, this aim is accomplished by foregrounding rather than disguising the technologies of representation themselves. *Andromeda*'s extensive use of split-screen composition exemplifies this strategy, as the technique highlights the process of producing the image by drawing attention to the usually invisible effects of framing the shot. *The Andromeda Strain* further emphasizes the gap between the audio and visual tracks of the film by fetishizing the scientific technologies of vision that enable the search for the invisible contaminant. In the process, the film also fetishizes the body of the central male protagonist, the "odd man," who ends up functioning as both subject and object of medical investigation.[5]

In keeping with the public health films discussed in earlier chapters, *Andromeda* painstakingly frames its fictional narrative as a purely documentary presentation of a historical event, while simultaneously relying upon futuristic imaging technologies to provide the film's aura of scientific authenticity. But while earlier public health films aimed to train viewers in identifying and thus avoiding possible scenarios of contamination, this film disavows the notion that contagion can be spatially or demographically isolated. Detached from individual bodies and dislodged from geographical locales, the representation of contagion in *Andromeda* is aligned with the technologies of globalization that enable widespread belief in scientific authority in the post-war period. Modernized (even extraplanetary) technologies of transportation and communication bring contagion, not progress, and high-tech modes of visualizing invisible pathogens enable the further entanglement of the discourse of contagion with advanced imaging systems. The technologies of representation used in this film eliminate the previous gap between documentary and nondocumentary modes of depicting disease that had characterized public health films through the 1950s. This strategy enacts the fantasy that internalized surveillance will make invisible contagions visible by eliminating the gap between documentary and "new media," thus flawlessly joining the visible and the invisible. By closing this gap, *The Andromeda Strain* participates in the historical transformation of visual representations of invisible contagions, which reaches its apotheosis with the development of digital imaging technologies that can convincingly integrate authentic and simulated or indexical and artificial modes of representation, as in the film *Outbreak*, which I will discuss later in this chapter. And yet, the ultimate goal of world health, to visualize invisible contagions, remains unmet.

DOCUMENTING CONSPIRACY: *THE ANDROMEDA STRAIN*

The Andromeda Strain presents itself as a documentary account of the discovery of an unidentified, highly contagious, and deadly infectious agent in a small desert town in the southwestern United States. The crashed satellite that is the source of contagion is investigated by a team of top-secret scientists in a high-tech, underground laboratory (the "Wildfire" lab), while above ground, government officials debate whether to drop a nuclear bomb on the site of contamination. The opening title sequence of the film announces its documentary mode of discourse by suggesting the immediacy of the story's temporality (as if the camera were present for the unfolding of these historical events) and invoking the potential sensitivity and contemporary relevance of the events recounted in the film. By treating the film as a collection of "documents," the narration of *The Andromeda Strain* self-consciously adopts an epistemological position at the intersection of science and fiction—a site that will later become central to, though also obscured by, the development of digital media. As we have seen, the attempts to separate cinematic pleasure and instruction through film censorship regulations did lead to the separation of exhibition venues, but this also resulted in the interweaving (not opposition) of scientific and fictional representational techniques. *The Andromeda Strain*'s fascination with documenting the presence of contagion is demonstrated by its obsessively realist approach to representing the project as an authentic scientific experiment of enormous geopolitical import. Consider the film's opening intertitle: "Acknowledgments: This film concerns the four-day history of a major American scientific crisis. We received the generous help of many people attached to Project Scoop at Vandenberg Air Force Base and the Wildfire Laboratory in Flatrock, Nevada. They encouraged us to tell the story accurately and in detail. The documents presented here are soon to be made public. They do not in any way jeopardize the national security."

Immediately following this disclaimer, additional titles flash onscreen in rapid sequence, undercutting the truth value of the prior claim, but in doing so, enhancing the film's own claims to documentary authenticity: "This document contains information affecting the national defense of the United States, within the meaning of the Espionage Laws, Title 18, U.S.C. Sections 793 and 794, the transmission or revelation of which in any manner to an unauthorized person is prohibited by law." This warning is followed by an ostensibly top-secret map of the west coast of the United States, menacingly titled "Biowar Map." In setting up the tension between the indexical and the artificial, truth and secrecy, the opening credits sequence of *The Andromeda Strain* not only sets up the film's plot but also sets the dialectic of visibility and invisibility in motion through the structure of conspiracy.

In strictly scientific fashion, this film's chronological account of the crisis is divided into four units, titled "First Day," "Second Day," and so forth. The film's temporality is further broken down through the use of television news-style subtitles, noting the exact location and precise time of day that each segment occurred. This device simultaneously invests the film with televisual "liveness" and enhances its authority as a retrospective account of "what really happened."[6] But *Andromeda*'s documentary status is challenged by the problem of capturing an indexical representation of "reality," particularly in the face of a highly sensitive government coverup. This tension is articulated here through the cinematic equivalent of the conspiracy theory's "crisis of signification"; the destabilization of the referent that characterizes the narrative of conspiracy is expressed cinematically through a disjunction between the audio and visual tracks of the film. The frictions between *Andromeda's* different discursive layers are generated through a proliferation of imaging technologies. So many different versions of the "truth" are generated with the assistance of the all-powerful computer that runs the Wildfire lab that it becomes impossible to distinguish genuine scientific discovery from over-determined effects intentionally generated by the government conspiracy. As the possibility emerges that the seemingly haphazard events chronicled by the film are in fact the effects of a government project to develop biological weapons, the increasingly intricate mapping of the virus becomes utterly vital in the search for the truth and utterly irrelevant, given the all-encompassing nature of the conspiracy.

During "Day One" of the film, a pair of soldiers from the nearby Vandenberg Air Force Base are sent into Piedmont, New Mexico, to recover the crashed satellite (a technology of global transportation and communication), only to discover that the entire population of the town is dead. Despite the seemingly graphic and visually arresting nature of the soldiers' discovery (suggested by their horrified exclamations over the radio), the entire sequence is shot from inside the Air Force Base command center. The transmissions from the rescue mission are broadcast over loudspeakers, visually represented only by close-ups of lines on a voice-wave monitor. By introducing the event that propels the film's pursuit of an indexical image of contagion through the audio track of the film, without accompanying visual images, this sequence establishes the film's linkage of contagion paranoia with a destabilization of semiotic registers. This breakdown of presumptively transparent communication hints at the fragmentation of subjectivity that Lacanian psychoanalytic theory has described as an effect of the entry into language, the symbolic order constituted through the gap between signifier and signified.[7] When it is linked to the fear of male bodily penetration later in the film, this fragmentation of subjectivity takes the form of a homosexual panic.[8]

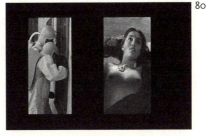

Once we finally do see the carnage that has been aurally represented, it is visually mediated and dissected through imaging technologies such as infrared, reverse-field film footage shot from a military plane taking reconnaissance photographs from the safe distance of the aerial long shot. The severity of the situation that is conveyed by these images prompts a second rescue mission to enter the town, but this time it consists of a scientist (Stone) and doctor (Hall) from the top-secret "Wildfire" mission, who are encased within protective biohazard spacesuits that will prevent the viral penetration that had caused the demise of the earlier satellite recovery team. During their exploration of the decimated town, the two investigators find countless corpses, seemingly stricken in mid-stride (the bodies are found in the acts of pumping gas, having a haircut at the barbershop, and so forth). In the midst of this display, the onscreen image suddenly splits in two, and as the investigators are shown peering through windows, the dead bodies they see are displayed in a series of disjointed close-ups on the other half of the screen, over a menacing musical soundtrack that jarringly lacks any dialogue (figure 80).

This voyeuristic sequence concludes with an image of a naked woman's breasts—the camera zooms in on the shot until it occupies the entire screen, reintegrating the two halves of the split image. The gratuitous quality of this shot seems incongruous in the context of the coldly scientific, clipped, and functionalist economy of the film's narration up to this point. But the seemingly unmotivated shot in fact reveals the film's fundamental epistemology. By sexualizing the search for the source of contagion, the shot effectively sexualizes the film's source of knowledge: the epidemiological gaze. However, as signaled by the further severance of the audio and visual tracks of the film, this is an anxious, not pleasurable form of sexualized gaze. The

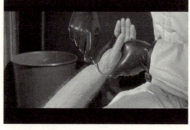

The Andromeda Strain (1971)

underlying significance of this morbidly voyeuristic visual excess is revealed when the investigators discover the missing satellite inside of the local doctor's office. While Stone examines the satellite itself, Hall inexplicably busies himself with unfastening the doctor's belt, removing him from the chair in which he died, and pulling down his pants. When Hall proudly displays his findings, Stone refuses to look at the doctor's bared buttocks—assuming that Hall is playing an infantile prank, Stone scolds him, saying, "That's not funny!" It turns out that Hall has made a medical discovery and is attempting to convey that the man's blood has not pooled in the lowest extremity, as it would have in a normal cadaver. While the doctor's backside is not revealed onscreen, Hall's subsequent actions suggest the psychological consequences of his experience of epiphany upon gazing at another man's naked body: he slits the doctor's wrist, and we see, in close-up, the crystallized blood that pours from the cut (figure 81).[9]

Following the logic of contagion that Eve Sedgwick has attributed to the reaction formation of "homosexual panic," the notion that a fellow doctor's exposed genitals could be the source of scientific revelation contaminates Hall's own body later in the film, when his naked form becomes the object of the scientifically sexualized gaze.[10] During the extended bodily examination and disinfection sequence that follows the Wildfire team's arrival at the top-secret underground laboratory, Hall's naked body is featured as the central spectacle, which along with the futuristic investigative apparatus itself, is a key source of visual pleasure for the film. Significantly, Hall's body is displayed more frequently than any other, including that of the sole female member of the team. It is clearly Hall, not the tough, sarcastic, and masculine Ruth, who is coded as an object of desire, the object "to-be-looked-at," and the implicit homoeroticism and consequent anxiety produced by this coding pervade the public health and science fiction films that represent contagion as male bodily penetration.

The bodily investigation sequence is intercut with scenes taking place in a location identified by subtitle as "White House Situation Room 2:40 P.M. E.S.T." There, a group of high-ranking officials debates whether or not Piedmont should be annihilated with a nuclear bomb. Images of topographical maps marking the contaminated area cover the room's walls, highlighting the threat of global contagion if the decision to drop the bomb is delayed. The interjection of cartography at this point metonymically links the threat of male bodily penetration with the threat of national penetration, absorbing both into the narrative of conspiracy, and the underlying paranoia of this linkage is further elaborated in flashbacks and flash-forwards, interspersed throughout the film, of senate hearings to justify the development of the Wildfire lab, and later to account for the events of the film's "four-day crisis." The skeptical and distanced posture of the previously enthusiastic senators in the flash-forwards confirms the conspiracy and cover-up that had only been hinted at thus far in the film. Such scenarios of official denial of the events laid out in the preceding collection of cinematic "documents" rapidly become iconographic in conspiracy films of the 1970s, functioning as a self-consciously weak form of narrative closure that highlights the epistemological impossibility of a conclusive utterance, given the radical gap between signifier and signified that seems only to produce "endless semiosis."[11] In fact, on the fourth day of the "crisis," when one of the scientists begins to suspect that Project Scoop (the military project that launched the satellite) was actually designed to produce a biological weapon, the team leader and liaison between the scientists and the government irritably dismisses the suggestion as paranoia.

The importance of bodily investigation to the narration of conspiracy is highlighted by the film's return to the Wildfire lab, where we see the naked backs of the three male team members pass through a sliding door marked "Exit to Decontamination & Immunization." The ensuing sequence displays a fascinating array of visual representations of the invisible features of these bodies: their figures are rendered as blurred bluish skeletal X-rays and magnetically manipulated heat-sensor images during radiation decontamination, and while their own bodily interiors are exposed to the camera,

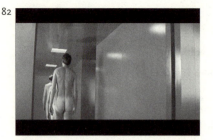

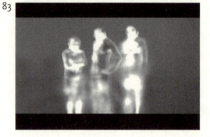

The Andromeda Strain (1971)

the group discusses their plans for investigating the organism in the satellite (figures 82 and 83). The contrast between the complete and thorough
mapping of the male bodies and their own utter lack of information about
the highly infectious agent they have been summoned to investigate posits
the two sets of organisms as the epistemological extremes within the scientific project of bodily exploration. As the group moves through progres-
sively more invasive levels of the disinfection process, the team leader tells
them, "We face quite a problem: how to disinfect the human body—one of
the dirtiest things in the known universe." The notion that human bodies
are inherently contaminated and must therefore be subjected to rigorous investigation and analysis by the automated examination apparatus, to identify
and eliminate the potential contagions lurking within, highlights the fantasy
of internalized surveillance that drives this film and, indeed, the discourse
of contagious globalization as a whole.

Subsequently, the team is sent into individual "body analysis" rooms,
and the camera follows Hall as he is directed by a sultry female voice on the
loudspeaker to arrange himself on an examination chair, legs spread, and
look into a round screen. The chair reclines as a blue ray passes over his
body, scanning for "fungal lesions" and various other impurities. An entranc-

ing array of abstract flashing colors fills the screen, hypnotizing Hall while a mechanical arm reaches down to inoculate him with "pneumatic injections of booster immunizations." That night, each team member except Hall is granted interiority through individualized split screen dream sequences. In contrast, the sexualized pleasure generated by Hall's submission to the aurally feminized "body analysis" machine is played out the next morning, when the same voice awakens Hall, and he attempts to engage "her" in flirtatious banter. The mechanized reply—"uncodable response"—is interrupted by a castigating male voice that intervenes over the loudspeaker, requesting that Hall "adopt a more serious attitude." Hall defends his "natural" desire by replying, "Sorry, her voice is quite luscious," in response to which the male voice of surveillance informs Hall that "she" is Miss Gladys Stevens, a sixty-three-year-old woman from Omaha who makes voice recordings for a living, thus effectively crushing Hall's fantasy of the feminized and therefore penetrable machine.[12] The linkage of the bodily probe with sexualized penetration is made even more explicit when, as the final step in purification, the team leader passes out anal suppositories for the scientists to complete the surveillance of their bodily interiors, and Ruth suggestively jokes, "Anyone care to join me for a smoke?"

Once the team finally passes through the decontamination procedure, the film's fascination with constructing visual images of the body's invisible interior shifts to the pathogenic organism itself. The search to locate the "Andromeda Strain" drives the rest of the film, through elaborate sequences of laboratory experiments that generate visuality by displacing the invisible contagion onto various lab animals whose exposure to the satellite produces observable bodily symptoms of infection as each specimen convulses and collapses on the floor of its cage. Revisiting the morbid fascination of the earlier split-screen sequence, the etiology of the Andromeda Strain is displayed through another split composition. Here, extreme close-ups of a monkey strapped to a lab table (receiving an intravenous injection from a contaminated rat) are intercut with close-ups of computer screens monitoring the animal's bodily functions, providing the scientifically objective perspective needed to determine the mode of contagion (airborne) and the "mechanism of death" (instantaneous crystallization of the blood). Once the organism is isolated, its representation becomes increasingly fragmented and mechanically manipulated: the computer screens that line the walls of the lab display an endless series of microscopic enlargements as well as streams of data dissecting and classifying the contaminant.

As noted above, *Andromeda*'s obsessive investigation of both the infectious agent and the male body that is positioned as the virus' most likely target functions through the classical Hollywood logic usually reserved for investigating the figure of the woman. But as Steve Neale has influentially observed, "In a heterosexual and patriarchal society, the male body cannot be marked explicitly as the erotic object of another male look: that look must be motivated in some other way, its erotic component repressed."[13] Just as the threatening pleasure of the woman's "lack" is conventionally punished through the voyeuristic and sadistic gaze, the threatening (homoerotic) pleasure of placing a male character in the position of visual spectacle in this film is punished by the threat of male bodily penetration by the virus.

But, as in the earlier public health and science fiction films, the fetishization of technologies of investigation and communication belies the anxiety about the parallel flows of information and contagion facilitated by these technologies. At several key moments throughout the film, the technology fails, threatening universal contagion. A simple mechanical error prevents the Wildfire team from receiving vital, time-sensitive wire transmissions about the scheduled atomic destruction of the town of Piedmont. The rapid regeneration of the virus overloads and crashes the lab computer, preventing further investigation into methods of containing or destroying the organism. And at the film's conclusion, the mutated and now harmless virus penetrates the lab's protective seal, prompting the computer's automatic self-destruct countdown, and the team cannot access the manual override because it is still under construction.

By painstakingly representing the impossibility of containing the "Andromeda Strain" within the infected town, or even within the high-tech underground government lab where most of the film's action takes place, *Andromeda* suggests the universality of the threat of infection. The entanglement of technophilia and homophobia in this film combines the anxieties about new media, globalization, and national and bodily contagion by invisible invaders that have characterized all of the films discussed in this book. But the abstraction of contagion in *The Andromeda Strain* is recorporealized with the advent of AIDS; in *Outbreak* and other AIDS-era contagion narratives, penetration anxiety is racialized through techniques that recall earlier public health films like *The Eternal Fight* (1948) and *The Silent Invader* (1957), but with a difference. The development of digital imaging technologies conclusively eliminates the gap between the visible and the invisible, the indexical and the artificial. Documentary footage and special effects are integrated into a cinematic mythology of total surveillance, but as with postwar public health films, the proliferation of images of contagion cannot make microscopic pathogens visible to the naked eye—it can only result in the proliferation of national and bodily penetration anxieties. But what explains this shift from embodiment to abstraction and then back to embodiment? Between the universalized abstraction of contagion in *Andromeda* and the digitized depiction of contagion in *Outbreak*, an important set of media representations are produced—AIDS educational videos. These films may enable us to understand the apparent contradiction of technologically sophisticated imaging systems being accompanied by historically regressive modes of representing contagion.

FROM ABSTRACTION TO EMBODIMENT:
HIV/AIDS EDUCATIONAL VIDEOS

Several important events took place in the realms of public health and mass media in the period between the conspiracy theory approach to contagion (typified by *Andromeda*) and the digital era (typified by *Outbreak*). As John Duffy has demonstrated, the widespread postwar faith in the powers of antibiotics and scientifically advanced medicine to eradicate contagious diseases led practitioners of public health to emphasize chronic and environmental diseases in the 1960s and 1970s. Writing in 1990, Duffy argued that "in the last forty years, as it became evident that industrial wastes were threatening our air, water, and food, public health authorities began to shift their emphasis from bacterial to physiochemical agents produced by industry."[14] This shift was reflected in public health films; relatively few films dealt with contagious disease until the AIDS crisis forced a return to earlier concerns. In the interim, three major developments created the conditions of possibility for the new public health films of the 1980s to treat issues of disease transmission in a more sophisticated manner than had previously been the case.

And yet, the movement away from the abstracted representation of contagion in the 1960s and 1970s ultimately leads to a paradoxical reassertion of the body in digitally enhanced representations of contagion in the 1990s, typified by the Hollywood film *Outbreak*.

The period between *Andromeda* and *Outbreak* is defined by the transformation of the regulation and content of Hollywood film, the emergence of videotape, and the subsequent shift to television as the primary medium of health education during the AIDS crisis. Just as the bacteriological revolution of the 1880s raised the possibility that medical and popular imaging of contagion would transcend the historical dependence on crude, stereotyped images of disease carriers as pathologized aliens (whether national, racial, or sexual), the changes in the fields of cinema and public health in this later period also raised the possibility of radical change. Ultimately, both of these potentially revolutionary moments went unfulfilled, but significant incremental change nonetheless occurred, and the boundaries defining the limits of the transformation contain important lessons about the relationships between educational media, entertainment, and sociocultural change.

Historians have chronicled the many transformations in the American film industry from World War Two to the present, but the key events for the purposes of this study were the *Paramount* decrees in 1948 and the *Miracle* decision in 1952. By dismantling the stranglehold of the vertically integrated monopolies of the studio system and granting motion pictures the protections of the First Amendment, these events led to the demise of the Hollywood studio system and the replacement of the Production Code with the ratings system in 1968, resulting in a radical expansion of the range of representational possibilities in mainstream, commercial cinema.[15] The most significant consequences of these changes for the broad field of representations comprising the discourse of world health were Hollywood's new permissiveness toward explicit representations of sex and the industry's newfound (if partial and temporary) sophistication in its treatment of racial themes. These topics had preoccupied film reform movements in the early twentieth century, and the restrictions that eventually governed their representation in film emphasized the potential for both moral and biological contagions that seemed to result from racial and sexual intermingling in the theaters and onscreen. Without these restrictions in place, one might imagine a filmic response to the AIDS crisis that was as radical a departure from the past as the blaxploitation movement was from *Guess Who's Coming to Dinner?* (1967).[16]

In fact, the comparison is not arbitrary—this set of films can productively illuminate the challenges facing AIDS-era public health film producers. As Ed Guerrero has argued, heightened race consciousness generated by the civil rights movement, "dissatisfaction with Hollywood's persistent degradation of African Americans," and the "near economic collapse of the film industry at the end of the 1960s" sparked the rise of a new genre that came to be known as "blaxploitation," originating with films like *Sweet Sweetback's Baadasssss Song* (1971) and *Shaft* (1971).[17] The enormous popularity of these films "forced Hollywood to respond to the rising expectations of African Americans by making black-oriented features," especially once it became clear that these films could potentially "solve the film industry's political and financial problems."[18] While numerous critics have identified the shortcomings of this potentially revolutionary movement,[19] the key point is that a set of films was produced that represented a powerful departure from the status quo, which seemed to prove that activism could indeed be effective, especially in periods of structural transformation in the mass media.

But Guerrero also argues that there was a backlash in the 1980s against the gains of blaxploitation. From the perspective of dominant culture, these films represented the acquisition of a mass media voice by a previously disenfranchised group, which gave rise to an ideologically conservative cycle of production Guerrero calls the "cinema of recuperation."[20] Thus, the 1980s were a period of backlash, when most of the positive gains in mass media representations of African Americans were lost. This argument suggests a cyclical theory of history and hegemony involving rebellion against negative images leading to a temporary phase of positive image production, followed by a reactionary phase of backlash that undermines most of the movement's gains.[21]

This model of backlash against racial minorities provides an important model for analyzing the public health films produced in response to the emerging AIDS crisis. As films that, like their predecessors, depended heavily on images of both racial and sexual "others" to define the boundaries of purity and danger,[22] AIDS education films might be seen as a test case not only for this theory of backlash but also for understanding the intersecting modes of representation in popular and scientific contexts—especially as the AIDS crisis is a period when the boundaries between those realms notably dissolve. Just as the early blaxploitation films can be seen as a reaction to the negative racial stereotypes that Hollywood had produced throughout its history, early activist AIDS videos can be seen as a reaction to the negative racial and sexual stereotypes that had long characterized mass media representations of gay men in general and that defined early network news coverage of the AIDS crisis in particular.

As James Kinsella and others have argued, early informational and educational programming on the epidemic represented predominantly white gay men, black Haitians, and Africans as the pathologized vectors of contagion.[23] In its most insidious form, the dominant mode of representation produced a general sense that AIDS was a deserved plague upon homosexuals and minorities—a horror to be sure, but one that only afflicted already stigmatized "others." In doing so, these television news programs and medical films drew upon the long history of associating racial and sexual "deviance" with threats to public health, as we have seen in the films discussed in earlier chapters. In fact, the notion that minority populations should be seen as the natural hosts of the worst diseases—the idea that there is an affinity between so-called degenerate biology and degenerative diseases—is so historically ingrained into commonsense understandings of contagion that the most typical phrasing of early panic about AIDS entailed sounding the alarm that the disease is *not* exclusively a gay, racial minority disease.

While initial coverage treated AIDS as frightening but distant, the discourse soon shifted to emphasize universal vulnerability. The need for precaution was often phrased in terms that highlighted the invisible privilege of invulnerability often assumed by white heterosexuals: "The AIDS virus is a threat to Americans in all walks of life. It is a sexually transmitted disease that does not discriminate between men and women, young and old, white and black," quoted in *AIDS: What You Need to Know* (1987). This warning is repeated almost verbatim in *The AIDS Movie* (1986), and in *The AIDS Antibody Test* (1987), as "The disease knows no sexual or racial boundaries." *AIDS: On the Front Line* (1987) argues, "AIDS kills—it doesn't discriminate. It's not who you are but what you do." Furthering this argument, *AIDS and Health-Care Workers: A Video Report* (1988) observes that, "We have learned that AIDS is no respecter of persons." Implicit in such statements is the assumption that there are diseases that *do* "respect" certain persons and discriminate against others, as well as a subtle sense of regret that unfortunately, AIDS is not one of them. The widespread expression of this warning in AIDS videos reveals just how commonplace is the idea that diseases are racially and sexually biased and, thus, highlights the extent to which the principles underlying the ideology of world health have come to define the most basic, historically entrenched and unconscious attitudes about health and disease.

In fact, this commonsense notion is so pervasive that it can also function in reverse—nonwhite people who are accustomed to being seen as the bearers of disease respond to AIDS in the same manner as privileged white commentators. In *Other Faces of AIDS* (1989), a gay black man admits that when he first started hearing about AIDS as a disease of gay white men, he thought, "Thank god it's them—it's always us. . . ." And this sentiment is repeated by a black heterosexual woman in . . . *Like Any Other Patient* (1989), who also confesses that before she was infected she always thought people with human immunodeficiency virus (HIV) were white and gay. But even while the early public health films on HIV and AIDS clearly stigmatized racial and sexual "others," a close examination of developments in the dominant mode of representing people with AIDS reveals that, over a relatively short period of time, these films self-consciously adjusted their depiction of the causes and consequences of the epidemic. Although the end result is still more than a little bit tinged with bias, this transformation nonetheless proves that the work of cultural critics and activists can indeed make a difference. The AIDS crisis represents a historically unique case of rapid, low budget production of videos that were highly responsive to the continually developing state of research on modes of transmission, testing, and treatment and that were also responsive to the critiques of AIDS activists who vocally condemned the racism and homophobia of the early films and television programs.[24] As a result of the need for constant adjustment of the research findings and educational content, these films were also able to adjust the form in which the message was delivered.

The rapidity and adaptability of the production process was partly an effect of the technological shift from film to the less expensive and more flexible medium of video as well as a shift from single-site exhibition to broadcasting. While videotape technology had been available since the late 1970s, it wasn't until the mid-1980s that the widespread use of videotape led to the demise of 16 mm educational filmmaking.[25] In addition, the incorporation of journalistic themes into entertainment programming on television in this period, especially in the form of newsmagazines, further shifted the focus from film to television as the primary source of educational information about health and hygiene. While reality programming would steadily increase until it came to dominate entertainment programming on network television in the 1990s, the subgenre of the informational television newsmagazine became especially popular in the 1980s.[26] A review of the key films and videos of the first decade of the AIDS epidemic reveals the importance of primetime television programming on the major commercial networks and the Public Broadcasting Service in generating awareness (and sometimes, misinformation) among the general public about the disease.

But perhaps most importantly, the discursive responsiveness of the mass media was largely generated in recognition of the corrective work of activist video collectives who replied directly to the inadequate (and often inaccurate) information that was available through mainstream sources.[27] One of the most significant and widespread adjustments was the discursive shift from emphasizing risk groups to emphasizing risk behaviors. Initially, AIDS videos shared the perspective of postwar public health films that warned viewers to avoid certain types of people and certain locations in order to avoid infection. In these films, demographic and geographic containment procedures advised that racial and sexual minority identities were the sources of contamination that should be avoided (if not quarantined).

The move toward "humanizing" people with AIDS led to a reversal of the process of abstraction described thus far, changing bodies into concrete individuals, rather than representative types. In . . . *Like Any Other Patient*, the narrator directly addresses the audience, telling us, "The point of this program is that we want you to see the people, not just the disease." The earliest HIV and AIDS videos perpetuated the representational techniques of postwar public health films, using typologies of gay men and intravenous drug users, Haitians, Africans, and sometimes prostitutes to displace panic over infection onto pathologized racial and sexual "others." These early videos were heavily criticized by activists and other advocates of people with AIDS, and this criticism had a discernable effect in transforming the quality of images of people with AIDS from the late 1980s and early 1990s to the present. While it is unfortunately impossible to claim a wholesale transformation in the mode of representing people with AIDS, the insistent emphasis on behavior over identity does create a discernible shift in tone, even when it is only a shift toward more inclusive stigmatization of all infected persons, regardless of their sexual identity, race, or the mode of HIV transmission.[28]

And yet, certain techniques in these films remind viewers of the continued concerns of public health with two key issues: the invisibility of contagion and the global processes that make this invisibility an ever-present threat. *Thumbs Up for Kids! AIDS Education* (1989) emphasizes the importance of imagining the presence of disease and thus making invisible germs visible by putting flour on the hands of children, who then touch objects and people around the room. The film uses this technique to demonstrate that unlike the cold germ—a skin germ—you can only get the "AIDS germ" from things that are inside of the body. But the reassurance that this technique might afford is easily undermined by films like *AIDS: Everything You and Your Family Need to Know . . . But Were Afraid to Ask* (1988), which reminds viewers of the threat posed by invisible infections: "About one third of people with AIDS will not have any visible symptoms." The problem is reiterated in *What You Should Know About AIDS* (1987): "You can't tell just by looking at a person." And this observation is followed up by emphasizing the official shift from earlier CDC categories of "risk groups" to "risky activities"—"it's not just who you are but what you do."

The familiar strategy of using an animated globe to highlight hotspots of disease is adapted to reveal hotspots of "homosexual activity" in *About AIDS* (1986), and this globe collapses racial and sexual "otherness" by tracing a line from Africa to Haiti to the United States, where cities with large gay communities are highlighted (figures 84 and 85). While the globe would seem to assure a certain kind of demographic isolation, the voiceover undermines this assurance, as it has in so many public health films since World War Two: "Because of the variety of infections from which people with AIDS suffer, the disease may show itself in many ways, and there is no single group of signs and symptoms by which it can be recognized." This threat is underscored by statistics on the invisibility of the disease: "It is estimated that for every

84

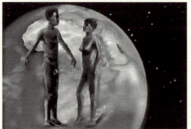

85

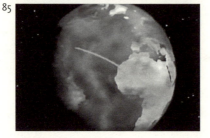

About AIDS (1986)

known case of AIDS, 50 to 100 people are infected with the virus." This video still focuses on high-risk groups—it hasn't yet made the shift to emphasizing high-risk behaviors, and in fact it clearly sees the spread of the disease as caused by a degenerate minority: "It is likely that the disease will spread from high-risk groups to the general population."[29]

In contrast, the radically democratizing potential of the AIDS crisis is highlighted in *AIDS Hits Home* (1986) when the narrator of the program, CBS anchor Dan Rather, points out that "The people who are dying look a lot like you and me." Later in the program, Rather further emphasizes the point: "AIDS is not a gay disease, AIDS is a venereal disease—it just happened to hit the gay population first." As a result of this discursive shift, invisibility surprisingly becomes the basis for arguing against discrimination, whereas in earlier films, invisibility essentially caused—or at least reinforced—discrimination, based on the argument that one had to look for observable signs of difference such as skin color or physiognomy to avoid contamination.

While the historical transformations that enabled the emergence of blaxploitation could have also allowed the development of different treatments of sexuality that engaged with issues of HIV and AIDS, they did not. Public health films and videos on television followed a trajectory from a form of abstraction akin to *Andromeda* to a more humanitarian form of embodiment, but this shift largely failed to transform the fictive modes of representing people with AIDS. Instead, commercial motion pictures tended to reproduce the homophobia and racism that AIDS activists had somewhat minimized in most public health films.[30] As Kylo-Patrick R. Hart argued in his book-length study, *The AIDS Movie*, most mainstream AIDS films "failed to adequately serve the needs of a wide range of audience members by ignoring the changing demographics of the AIDS pandemic and reinforcing the stigma associated with homosexuality in American society, as well as the perception of AIDS as a disease perpetuated almost exclusively by gay men, among other undesirable social outcomes."[31] In other words, the transformation of educational films accomplished by AIDS activists did not carry through to mainstream entertainment. But while films that are explicitly about AIDS are important to the discourse of world health as a whole, films about contagious globalization provide especially fascinating examples of how the dialectic of indexicality and artificiality has (and has not) changed over time—for a more recent example, we now turn to *Outbreak*.

"THE PUCKER FACTOR"

Recent contagion films are distinguished from postwar public health films by their ability to use new digital imaging technologies to give form to previously unrepresentable, invisible contagions. And yet, in many of these films, the latest cinematic visualization techniques serve not to revise, but rather to reinforce the conflation of disease and bodily difference. In *Outbreak* (1995), medical penetration is collapsed with viral penetration as technologies of representation become both cause and cure of (homo)sexual contagion. Despite its enhanced ability to visualize the invisible, *Outbreak* traces an epidemiological path whose global scope is conveyed through a racialized and sexualized narrative of the "African AIDS" epidemic (though here the disease is called "Motaba"). Because *Outbreak* combines an emphasis on technologies of representation and a preoccupation with bodily boundaries, the film can be seen as a culmination of the developments in the discourse of world health discussed in previous chapters. In this film, national and bodily borders are invaded by a global contagion carried by racially and sexually "deviant" bodies, whose actions are framed within a narrative of conspiracy.

Moreover, the flow of contagion is visualized through the now familiar dialectic of indexicality and artificiality. However, the "artificial" representational techniques employed in *Outbreak* no longer suffer from the inadequacies of the more rudimentary animation and special effects that abruptly severed the diegetic coherence of earlier public health and science fiction films. The digital imaging technologies used in this more recent film seamlessly integrate the indexical and the artificial, thus fulfilling the world health fantasy of visualizing invisible contagions in everyday life. As my discussion of *Outbreak* will demonstrate, the feared penetration of national and bodily borders that has characterized the discourse of world health since its inception is thoroughly reified in popular cultural imagery of AIDS. While my discussion of *Hospital Sepsis* and *The Andromeda Strain* demonstrated a movement toward the abstraction of contagion, here we see a reembodiment of contagion that is continuous with the imaging techniques of AIDS videos, but is particularly striking given the simultaneous abstraction of the vector of contagion through the rhetoric of electronic viruses.[32]

The discursive prevalence of viral disease (such as mad cow disease, severe acute respiratory distress syndrome, Eastern equine encephalitis), epidemics, and invasions in the news media is paralleled in popular culture with the recent videogame, *Biohazard Outbreak*; films such as the remake of *Dawn of the Dead* (2004), *28 Days Later . . .* (2002), *Twelve Monkeys* (1995), *Hackers* (1995), *Mimic* (1997), *Virus* (1999), *Mission: Impossible II* (2000); television series like *Dark Skies*, *The X Files*, *Roswell*, and *Alien Nation*; and made-for-TV movies such as *Runaway Virus* (2000), *Pandora's Clock* (1996), and *The Stand* (1994), not to mention the explosion of fictional and nonfictional journalistic "disease detective" exposés on the topic. The shelves of popular and academic bookstores are filled with such recent titles as *Virus X: Tracking the New Killer Plagues* (1998); *Viruses, Plagues and History* (1998); *Plague Time: How Stealth Infections Cause Cancers, Heart Disease, and Other Deadly Ailments* (2000); *The Devil's Flu: The World's Deadliest Influenza Epidemic and the Scientific Hunt for the Virus that Caused It* (2000); *Flu: The Story of the Great Influenza Pandemic of 1918 and the Search for the Virus that Caused It* (1999); *The Invisible Enemy: A Natural History of Viruses* (2000); *Biography of a Germ* (2000); *Anthrax: The Investigation of a Deadly Outbreak* (1999); the Pulitzer Prize–winning *Guns, Germs, and Steel: The Fates of Human Soci-*

eties (1997); not to mention the best-selling *The Hot Zone* (1994), *The Coming Plague* (1994), and the numerous medical thrillers by Robin Cook, including *Outbreak* (1987).[33]

Richard Preston, author of *The Hot Zone*, attempted to explain the popular and scientific attention to contagion in a *Newsweek* interview promoting the publication of his book, which coincided with the 1995 Ebola outbreak in Zaire:

> NEWSWEEK. Why are people so fascinated by viruses these days?
>
> PRESTON. There's a deep curiosity, there's a sense of horror. And also I think that in the backs of people's minds, ever present, is the AIDS virus.
>
> NEWSWEEK. With all the books, movies, and television shows, is this country in the midst of a sort of viral fad? Have we crossed the line from news stories to deadly viruses as entertainment?
>
> PRESTON. What's happening in Zaire is only too real. All the popular stuff, including "The Hot Zone" and the movies, are a reflection of a kind of geological shift in scientific perceptions about what's happening biologically to the human species. There's a perception that we face unprecedented threats from new, emerging infectious diseases. Popularization is a very good thing.[34]

As my earlier discussion of the "bacteriological revolution" of the 1880s has shown, these supposedly "unprecedented threats" are in fact far from new. But the discursive intersections of global telecommunications and global contagion have exaggerated the sense of temporal as well as spatial reduction of distances between global outbreaks and local infestations, resulting in a heightened perception of the omnipresence of contagion and producing these most recent expressions of "penetration panic."

The primary question in media coverage of the May 1995 Ebola outbreak in Kikwit, Zaire (now Congo), concerned the stability of national boundaries; everyone wanted to know whether the virus would spread to the rest of the world. Detailed accounts of the horrors of the African plague collapsed the contaminated body with the diseased nation-state, in diametric opposition to the "noninfected but infectible" national body of the United States. The obsessive repetition of the question—"will it spread?"—belied a widespread fear of global contagion, familiar since the postwar era but currently renewed in the discourse of AIDS. Accompanying this question was the unstable image of a coherent and impregnable national body that was persistently foregrounded through statements that emphasized the disintegrating boundaries between local and global, such as, "The presence of international airports puts every virus on earth within a day's flying time of the United States."[35] As we have seen, such statements have characterized the rhetoric of world health since (at least) the 1930s, but the historical simultaneity of the AIDS crisis and the emergence of new media technologies that invisibly entwine even the farthest reaches of the globe in a network of commerce and contamination has invested the discourse of contagion with an enhanced sense of urgency, if not panic.

By linking "African" racial geography with degeneracy and disease, the popular representations of the Ebola outbreak mimicked the very epidemic they described, spreading racialized contagion-phobia and penetration panic through the networks of information and entertainment that collectively constitute the realm of popular culture.[36] In a June 1995 report on the Ebola outbreak in Zaire, an *NBC Nightly News* story narrated by Tom Brokaw featured clips from the Hollywood films *And The Band Played On* (1993) and *Outbreak* (1995) to visually represent the current crisis. The images depicted actors playing space-suited Biosafety Level 4 CDC and USAMRIID (United States Army Medical Research Institute of Infectious Diseases) teams, exploring infected African villages. The newscast made no verbal mention of the origins or fictive nature of the film segments, identifying their nondocumentary source only briefly in the subtitle noting the image credits. This seamless integration of fictional and nonfictional accounts of the spread of disease typifies the discourse of contagious globalization in the digital era. While earlier accounts of such an outbreak would have oscillated between documentary footage and animation, leaving an obvious (and ontological) gap between the indexical and artificial modes of representation, contemporary technological advances have facilitated the slippage between the authentic and the simulation. Thus, any combination of fictional and nonfictional images and sounds can equally signify as "real" or "fake," depending on the representational context. The slippage from indexical to artificial representations of the invisible poses a unique problem when the global flow of contagion is confronted with national and bodily borders. The world health formula of "visualization equals inoculation" requires that disease be attached to concrete, identifiable vectors of contagion. Consequently, the chain of infection produced by the cinema of world health prioritizes visuality over "authenticity," and this displacement results in the conflation of racial and sexual difference with disease in the representation of the Ebola virus.

The emergence of Ebola into the popular discourse of contagion in the United States can be dated from the publication of Richard Preston's article, "Crisis in the Hot Zone," in the October 26, 1992, issue of *The New Yorker* magazine. This article describes both the discovery of the Ebola virus in a 1976 outbreak (which killed 274 people in the village of Yambuku, Zaire)[37] and the even more sensationalized story of the 1989 appearance of a new strain of the virus within U.S. borders, in monkeys at the Primate Quarantine Unit of Hazelton Research Products (a division of Corning Incorporated). As described by the *New York Times*, the article was "the true story of a United States Army biological strike team's race to stop one of the world's deadliest—and most infectious—viruses from escaping a medical lab in Frederick, MD, and spreading into a major city."[38] Hollywood studios began a bidding war over the article within twenty-four hours of its release.[39] The article was expanded into the 1994 best seller, *The Hot Zone*, which loosely provided the basis for the movie *Outbreak*.

These cultural productions repeatedly articulate the fantasy of a temporal and spatial evolutionary gap between modern and "premodern" worlds, even as geopolitical and subjective boundaries continually dissolve in the contemporary "borderless" world. Consider the following passage from *The Hot Zone*, which describes the ruminations of Colonel C. J. Peters, MD, Chief of the Disease Assessment Division at USAMRIID in Fort Detrick, Maryland, and overall leader of the Reston biohazard operation:

> He wondered about AIDS. What would have happened if someone had noticed AIDS when it first began to spread? It had appeared without warning, secretly, and by the time we noticed it, it was too late. If only we had had the right kind of research station in central Africa during the nineteen-seventies . . . we might have seen it hatching from the forest. If only we had seen it coming . . . we might have been able to stop it,

or at least slow it down; . . . we might have been able to save at least a hundred million lives. . . . On the other hand, suppose AIDS had been noticed? Any "realistic" review of the AIDS virus when it was first appearing in Africa would probably have led experts and government officials to conclude that the virus was of little significance for human health and that scarce research funds should not be allocated to it—after all, it was just a virus that infected a handful of Africans, and all it did was suppress their immune systems. So what?[40]

The elusive origins of HIV parallel the elusive indexicality of AIDS; the fact that AIDS is not an identifiable "thing-in-itself" with a coherent and consistent set of symptoms has posed challenges for visual representation. The threat of contagion has come to signify through a series of metonymic displacements, in addition to racial and sexual difference: biohazard spacesuits, latex, and other prophylactics designed to prevent the penetration of vulnerable bodily boundaries.[41] In *Hemolytic Streptococcus Control*, the excessive proximity of male bodies to each other functioned as a sign of contamination; in *The Eternal Fight*, a visual montage of nonwhite faces marked the spread of disease. In *Outbreak*, race and sexuality are combined in the metonymic chain that fuses the iconography of "Africa" and "virus" by visually conflating a monkey and a "witch doctor" and then shifting from racial to sexual deviance once the virus enters U.S. borders.

This racialized imagery of contagion posits a teleological progression from the diseased "premodern" world to the modern, sanitized "First World," under increasing threat of infection in a historical period characterized by fluid national boundaries and transnational bodily movement. The foregrounding of racialized nationality in the Ebola discourse displaces the most recent articulation of disease and difference—American domestic AIDS phobia—onto the idea of "Africa." Thus, the fear of national and bodily invasion by invisible contagions is dispelled by visualizing the threat in the form of a racially and sexually marked body with spatially and temporally distant origins. But, as with the earlier public health films, the discourse of world health continues to be driven by anxiety over just how impermeable those national and bodily boundaries really are.

Outbreak's visual obsession with bodily integrity and technologies of disease surveillance results in obsessive intercutting between the phallic virus and scenarios producing a unique form of penetration panic. In a revision of the postwar public health films, alien invasion films, and conspiracy films discussed thus far, *Outbreak* and *The Hot Zone* express this fear not only by displacing the contagion onto nonnormative bodies but also by attributing consciousness and volition to a phallically anthropomorphized virus: "If you want to shake hands with one of these viruses, you had better wear a space suit." "That may be one of Ebola's strategies for success." "Look at this honker. Look at this long sucker here." "The walls were plastered with photographs of the Ebola virus. Some of the viruses were ten inches long and resembled ballpark frankfurters."[42] This conception of the phallic agency of Ebola produces a critically important trope in *The Hot Zone*: "the pucker factor." Preston's use of this term exemplifies the entanglement of racial and sexual "otherness" (to the normative white, heterosexual male) in the audiovisual discourse of world health, and its recent instantiation in the AIDS and Ebola discourse. Consider the following quotes from *The Hot Zone*: "It looked real. It felt real. He experienced what he would later describe as 'a major pucker factor' setting in. (This is a military slang term that refers to a certain tightening sensation in the nether regions of the body, in response to fear.)"[43] And later, "C.J. then gave an overview of the situation, telling the general about the monkeys in Reston, and finishing with these words: 'I'd say we have a major pucker factor about the virus in those monkeys. . . . We have to be very concerned and very puckered if it is of the same ilk as Ebola.' They had to be very puckered, Russell agreed."[44]

By linking the fear of penetration by a deadly virus with anal "puckering," this passage conflates the fear of anal penetration with death, thus collapsing the terms for representing "homosexual panic" and Ebola phobia. This frantic emphasis on boundary maintenance is articulated at the level of the body through descriptions of the horrifying porousness of Ebola-induced hemorrhagic fever, and at the national level, with the continual return to that most pressing question: could it happen here?

The virus seemed about to start an explosive chain of lethal transmission in Kinshasa, a poor, crowded city with a population of two million where the virus might go off like a bonfire. This epidemiological possibility triggered a panic in European capitals. Kinshasa has direct air links to Europe, and European governments contemplated blocking flights from Kinshasa . . . The Zairian government ordered its army to seal off the Bumba Zone with roadblocks, and all radio contact with the province was lost. Bumba had dropped off the earth, into the silent heart of darkness.[45]

It is precisely this threatened return of the colonial repressed through viral penetration of u.s. territory that invests these texts with a tone of desperate paranoia and hints at a conspiracy theory based on the malevolent "primitivism" attributed to the virus. By emphasizing the gap between "First" and "Third" worlds, the tension is simultaneously heightened and contained; the possibility of the virus "jumping species" threatens the terror of boundary dissolution, while the "evolutionary" division between species reassures the unlikelihood of such a jump.[46] The problem for a domestic outbreak, then, is to detect the diseased impostor, whose perverted American masquerade puts the entire nation at risk. As with earlier articulations of the discourse of contagious globalization, the key defensive tactic is to make the invisible menace visible. *Outbreak* attempts to accomplish this aim by obsessively producing visual representations of the invisible virus, thus rendering the threat of penetration effectively impotent; the film compulsively maps out the chain of contagion in order to dispel the fear that disease is everywhere and no one is safe. Thus, epidemiological mapping functions as viral countersurveillance; the anthropomorphized virus may have mounted an international conspiracy aimed at penetration of u.s. borders, but by obsessively representing the hypothetical geographic and demographic locations of the virus, health surveillance organizations can prevent the dissolution of national boundaries.

The coding of the spatio-temporal evolutionary divide as racial difference in *Outbreak* establishes a fantasized barrier to penetration of United States borders by infectious disease. When the USAMRIID team flies into Zaire to inspect the "present day" outbreak, the entry into the primordial hot zone is established through a cut from the interior of the high-tech helicopter to a medium-shot of a "witch doctor" bent over a mat strewn with ritual objects, who gazes suspiciously at the helicopter as it passes. Thus, before the threat of permeable national borders is explicitly raised in the film, certain visual

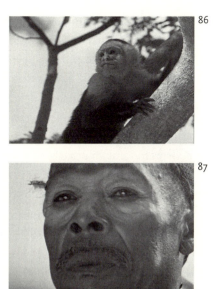

Outbreak (1995)

associations are established in the effort to fortify those boundaries. The hot zone sequence assures that if difference is not maintained through national borders, it will be maintained by evolutionary borders, as signaled through the cut to the primitive witch doctor. When the USAMRIID helicopters are leaving the village, having examined the diseased and dying black bodies found there, the camera again cuts from the interior of the helicopter to a medium-shot of a screeching monkey, then dissolves through a smoky mist to a close-up of the witch doctor's face, thus creating a visual metonymy linking monkey, black skin, and African "premodernity," as the vectors of an uncivilized and deadly contagion (figures 86 and 87).

The threat of national and bodily invasion by an invisible enemy is thus allayed, in part, by visualizing contagion on the surface of the body; "dark" racial marking makes disease detectable by the naked eye.[47] This anxiety is further articulated through *Outbreak*'s emphasis on visual technologies of surveillance and epidemiological mapping. Racial difference establishes the outside of the nation, limiting its terrain and localizing the potentially global scale of contagion. In contrast, sexual deviance functions as the invisible enemy within (alternately the passing homosexual or communist or alien), whose degeneracy threatens not only himself, but also a heterosexual couple, a research team, and ultimately, national security. The sexual threat is contained through the investigation of the diseased body with high-tech imaging devices; the omniscient epidemiological gaze serves as a counterpoint to the infectious transgressions of the figure who willingly opens his body to "viral" penetration.

The character of Casey (a principle member of the USAMRIID Biolevel 4 team) is coded as sexually deviant through his flagrant invulnerability to (or perhaps more appropriately, his "tolerance" for) the penetration panic that consumes the rest of the health surveillance team. He jokes sarcastically during tense moments in the film (including before and after witnessing a village bloodily devastated by "Motaba," the film's version of Ebola), he tosses glass vials around in the Biosafety Level 4 laboratory, pretending they are bottles of perfume, and he even tells jokes on his deathbed.[48] The consequences of Casey's social and sexual deviance are revealed later in the film when he becomes infected with Motaba. By functioning as a repository for the deadly virus and then infecting an innocent heterosexual woman, Casey becomes the locus of displaced contagion anxieties. Because he is infected through his own carelessness (falling asleep in the hazardous environment of the lab, ignoring his body's "natural" demands for sleep), and then keeps his infection a secret, Casey functions in the logic of *Outbreak* as a double for the "homosexual menace" of the AIDS crisis (the gay man who "chooses" to have unsafe sex and then "chooses" to infect other people with HIV).

The opposition of innocent heterosexuality to derelict homosexuality is underscored in a scene where Casey's deadliness is unmistakably fused with his status as a gay man—a "friend of Dorothy." As Casey awakens from a Motaba-induced coma, he murmurs to Sam (the leader of the USAMRIID team), "I had a wonderful dream, Auntie Em. You were there, you were there." This reference to a famous line spoken by the actress Judy Garland—a Stonewall-era gay cultural icon—at the end of *The Wizard of Oz* clearly codes the diseased Casey as a gay man dying of AIDS.[49] Moreover, as we discover later in the film, the infected monkey that brought the disease into the United States was smuggled across national borders illegally by an Asian sailor, whose unsanctioned intimacy with the contaminated creature is demonstrated not only by the man's death from Motaba, but also by the Polaroid photograph of the animal tucked into the springs of the overhead bunk in the ship's sleeping quarters, where most of his shipmates had pictures of their (human) female sweethearts. Thus homosexuality, racial difference, and deadly perversion are fused in the film's association of infection with the unnatural union between a human and an African monkey.[50]

"APPARENTLY THEY ALL GOT IT AT A MOVIE THEATER"

But such reckless sexual promiscuity is disciplined by the disembodied epidemiological gaze; *Outbreak*'s use of digital point-of-view camerawork enacts the fantasy of inoculation through visual representation that continues to drive the audiovisual discourse of world health today. The film's preoccupation with mapping the epidemiology of the seemingly inexplicable Motaba outbreak in the small, isolated town of Cedar Creek is reminiscent of the compulsion to visually map the spread of invisible disease in earlier public health films. The anxious reiteration of epidemiological redemption, the repeated claim that "truth" can be ascertained and that the links in the causal chain of contagion can be mapped, invests the postwar films and, more recently, *Outbreak* with a desperate desire for an indexical image of contagion.

The problem of visuality is articulated in *Outbreak* through two key representational techniques: the extensive use of point-of-view camerawork, shot through the face masks of Biohazard protection suits, and technologically enhanced visual representation of the virus itself, in both diegetic and nondiegetic registers. The visualization of invisible contagion in *Outbreak* benefits from the digital imaging technologies that seamlessly integrate the profilmic and the postphotographic; in two key sequences, the invisible virus is made visible as it flows through the public spaces of the film, spreading its web of infection across the town of innocent Americans.

The alternately embodied and disembodied visual aesthetic of contagion in this film is epitomized by a series of sequences shot from the point of view of an apparently omniscient, abstracted, high-tech surveillance system. This imagery reinforces the binary opposition that the film struggles to maintain between "First" and "Third" worlds, between the United States and Africa, by associating advanced medicine and scientific superiority with control of the body under siege by the deadly virus. *Outbreak* borrows the rhetorical linkage of Western technological superiority and invulnerability to global contagions from the discourse of AIDS. In "Inventing 'African AIDS,'" Cindy

Patton elucidates the processes by which categories of race and sexuality are inextricably bound to the construction of national boundaries. Patton describes a discourse that exemplifies "the confusion of biology (here, a viral infection) with historical specificities (here, colonialist underdevelopment) in an attempt to describe not only a material, but more importantly, a cultural difference between pre- and post-industrial societies."[51]

This "cultural difference" rhetorically constructs African medicine as unsophisticated and ineffective, and, in the case of Ebola, this argument functions as a contradiction. On one hand, the discourse places blame for the outbreak and spread of the virus on "civilization": land development (destruction of the rain forests), environmental pollution, overpopulation, political corruption, and capitalist greed, exemplified by Zaire's (now deposed and deceased) President Mobutu Sese Seko. Significantly, these causes are not identified as effects of postcoloniality or Western imperialist exploitation of African land and bodies. On the other hand, these manifestations of modernity are praised as the advantages of a highly developed society (the United States) and thus as a source of medical technology that can detect and halt the spread of disease through the implementation of advanced safety precautions. The irony, of course, is that none of the sophisticated, First World scientists at the CDC or USAMRIID has been able to locate the natural host of the Ebola virus (nor the origins of HIV), despite extensive field and laboratory research, nor has a vaccine or treatment been devised for Ebola or HIV. And yet, discursively, Western science prevails.

In the opening credits sequence of *Outbreak* (after an African mercenary camp infected with Motaba is obliterated by an air vacuum bomb in 1967), the camera tours the USAMRIID laboratories, moving from Biolevel-1 to Biolevel-4 in a single long take. The Steadicam sequence is filmed from the perspective of a person with high-level security clearance, as indicated by direct address gestures to the camera from various checkpoint personnel; but the point of view is disembodied, dissolving through physical barriers such as doors and windows and gracefully avoiding collisions with the scientists rushing through the labs.

The simultaneous embodiment and abstraction of the medical gaze in this film parallels the cinematic treatment of the virus itself. In Africa, the virus is represented through the visually condensed trope of the "premod-

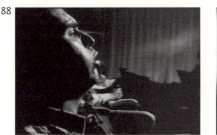

88

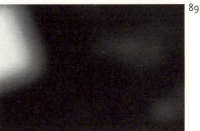

89

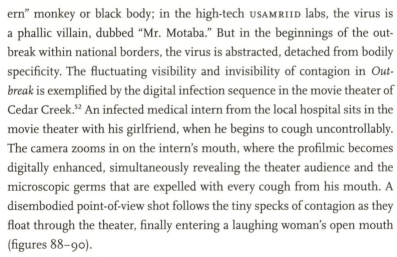

90

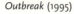

Outbreak (1995)

ern" monkey or black body; in the high-tech USAMRIID labs, the virus is a phallic villain, dubbed "Mr. Motaba." But in the beginnings of the outbreak within national borders, the virus is abstracted, detached from bodily specificity. The fluctuating visibility and invisibility of contagion in *Outbreak* is exemplified by the digital infection sequence in the movie theater of Cedar Creek.[52] An infected medical intern from the local hospital sits in the movie theater with his girlfriend, when he begins to cough uncontrollably. The camera zooms in on the intern's mouth, where the profilmic becomes digitally enhanced, simultaneously revealing the theater audience and the microscopic germs that are expelled with every cough from his mouth. A disembodied point-of-view shot follows the tiny specks of contagion as they float through the theater, finally entering a laughing woman's open mouth (figures 88–90).

The action in this sequence is both diegetic, in that the intern's germs are spread within the fictional world of the film and are central to the cause-effect chain of the narrative, and nondiegetic, in that the visual representation of those germs floating through the air is available to the viewing audience (and pointedly so, when screened in a movie theater), but not to the characters in the film. The choice of a movie theater as the public site of mass contagion not only exaggerates the paranoia already pervading this film; it also recalls the linkage of spectatorship and contagion in the education versus entertainment debates of the 1930s. The notion that film viewing could be as morally contaminating as the unhygienic environment of the dark and dirty theater itself drove reformers to demand regulation of motion picture content. *Outbreak* reiterates this threat, but with a difference. While the diegetic audience of uninformed spectators is indeed contaminated at the movie theater, the audience of *Outbreak* has the educational benefit of the digitally enhanced "contagion-cam." Having witnessed the seemingly indexical representation of the airborne pathogen, we can imagine the flow of contagion in the "real" movie theaters where we sit. However, as with the earlier public health films, this cinematic inoculation leads more easily to penetration panic than it does to a sense of hygienic security.

The blurring of diegetic and nondiegetic worlds also occurs in another crucial disease surveillance sequence, which takes place in the Cedar Creek hospital once the epidemic is fully underway. The hospital is overflowing with patients being tested and monitored by the USAMRIID and CDC teams, when a medic points out a patient that had been in the hospital for a week prior to the outbreak and "had no contact with anyone in isolation." The camera cuts to a close-up of the patient's face, covered with Motaba lesions. The soundtrack amplifies the rasp of Sam's breathing inside his spacesuit, and the camera cuts to a close-up of his face, as he looks around the room, then up at the ceiling. At this moment, the epidemiological gaze becomes a disembodied, digital point-of-view shot that zooms in on a close-up of the ceiling air vent, then dissolves through the metal grating, zooming inside to reveal the impossible perspective of the virus as it weaves through the curving air duct. Dissolving through another metal grate at the other end of the air duct, the camera reemerges into the profilmic in a new room, where Sam rushes in, looks up at the vent and then directly at the camera, declaring, "It's airborne!" (figures 91–95).

CONCLUSION

At a pivotal narrative moment in *Outbreak*, when the president's advisors are debating whether to approve "Operation Clean Sweep" (nuclear annihilation of the site of the outbreak), USAMRIID's General McClintock presents

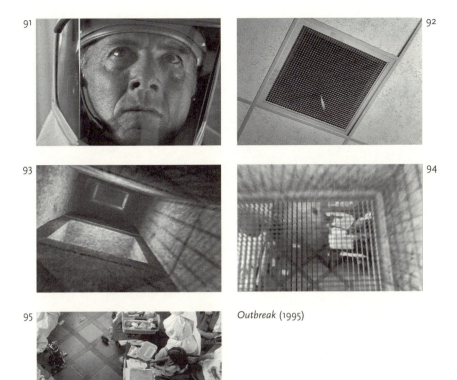

91

92

93

94

95

Outbreak (1995)

a computer map of the United States projected onto a screen, demonstrating the "predicted spread of contagion." This image is a digitally updated version of the map that appears in *The Fight Against the Communicable Diseases* (1950); the flow of contagion is indicated by waves of red, resembling a sea of blood that spreads from each coast, rapidly engulfing the entire country over a projected forty-eight-hour period (figures 96 and 97).[53] This computer simulation of the threat of global contagion is immediately legitimated by an indexical representation of the outbreak. The chief of staff tosses a pile of "documentary photographs" onto the conference table, demanding that everyone examine the visible evidence of the invisible contagion threatening national security: "Those are the citizens of Cedar Creek. Go on, look at

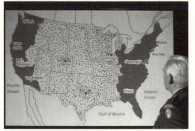

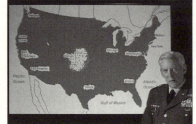

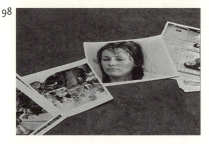

Outbreak (1995)

them. These are not statistics, ladies and gentlemen, they're flesh and blood. And I want you to burn those into your memories. Because those images should haunt us 'til the day we die." This declaration of the authenticity of the images is reiterated through a close-up shot of the photographs, displaying the dead bodies of Cedar Creek victims (figure 98). The "documentary" sequence cuts to a series of close-ups of bloody corpses being zipped into body bags by military personnel in protective spacesuits.[54]

The notion that the location of the virus can be pinpointed with electron-microscopic precision—as it is in *Outbreak*—would seem to fulfill the world health fantasy of total surveillance, and yet, the virus remains invisible to the naked eye. From this perspective, digital imaging is merely another technology of representation, like cinema, that can temporarily enhance the visual field but cannot fundamentally alter perception. And yet, digital imaging allows the artificial representation of contagion to be seamlessly integrated into the film, thus covering over the gap between the indexical and the artificial and thereby producing a compelling vision of internalized disease surveillance. Perhaps the production of such authentic simulations does amount to an altered form of perception after all. But if so, why is the trope of contagion still so anxiously reproduced in so many varied cultural forms? And if geopolitical and subjective boundaries are indeed dissolved in the global marketplace of postmodernity, why is the imagery of invasion still so prevalent in representations of the new media technologies that have enabled this "world without borders" to develop?

Whether "the invisible" is contagious disease or alien invasion, postwar media cultures strive to surpass the boundaries of visibility. Anxiously oscillating between the indexical and the artificial, the cinema of world health attempts to invest the filmed image with an authoritative form of realism through scientific surveillance and mastery of the public sphere and the private body. But the global benefits of hygienic modernization are not easily captured by audiovisual technologies of representation; documentary images can only reveal their truth through the assistance of special effects. Thus, scientific authority is generated through recourse to artificiality. And thus, the boundaries between the indexical and the artificial become impossible to identify. This representational problem has increasingly characterized the mass-mediated, image-based culture of global consumerism; the dialectic of visibility and invisibility that defines the project of world health raises the same questions about how to tell "truth" from "fiction" that now pervade the realm of digital imaging. The widespread use of "contagion" as a literal and figurative model for a variety of geopolitical and subjective transformations suggests that the project of world health defined a crucial ideological intersection in the postwar period. And as contemporary cultural productions attest, the impossibility of visually representing invisible contagions continues to propel the dialectic of world health and globalization today.

Conclusion

When we turn to computer viruses to consider a more recent example of technologies of transportation and communication being seen as purveyors of invisible contagion, we find that the elusiveness of the moment of digital infection is further exaggerated by the intangibility of the object under investigation. While the precise instant of contamination may be impossible to pin down in the postwar public health films discussed in earlier chapters, the site of infection was clearly identified as the human body (even as it was collapsed with a national body). But with computer viruses, the object becomes more elusive still—is it the computer itself? The wires that connect computers to each other? The abstract realm of cyberspace? The representations of the Internet in other media such as film, television, animation, print journalism, science fiction novels, or advertising? Mitsuhiro Yoshimoto has described cyberspace as an "object which does not exist anywhere except as an effect of its own image"[1] and one might say the same of contagion. Thus, there is a parallel between the fundamental unrepresentability of contagion and the unrepresentability of the Internet. And yet, the abstraction of the body into digital zeroes and ones on the Internet is belied by the insistent embodiment of the network through the rhetoric of disease and bodily difference.

The network news media coverage of the May 2000 Love Bug Internet virus that was ultimately traced to a computer hacker in the Philippines exemplifies this representational technique. The "premodern" geopolitical origins of the Love Bug both confirmed and disrupted Western expectations about the spread of contagious disease—a viral source in the "underdeveloped" world might be anticipated, but the potency of its threat to the (presumed) technological superiority of the West was not. The Love Bug thus occupies the same evolutionary discourse of globalization that, in the early-1980s, constructed "African AIDS" as evidence of the ongoing need for Western surveillance, regulation, and containment of previously colonized countries, by organizations like the WHO and the CDC.[2]

Moreover, the analytical framework applied to the Love Bug in mass media coverage borrowed from (and updated) the insidiously racialized rhetoric of many postwar public health films, such as *The Silent Invader*, that thematized contagion through anti-Asian xenophobic imagery, as in the following excerpt from *Time* magazine: "Like a real Asian influenza, the virus first emerged in Hong Kong. From there it spread westward with the sun, lying silently in wait in corporate email accounts until unsuspecting office denizens punched in, logged on and doubled-clicked on the file."[3]

The feared penetration of national and bodily borders that has characterized the discourse of world health since its inception is thoroughly reified in the convergent imagery of global computer viruses and the spread of HIV and AIDS; here we see a reembodiment of contagion that is particularly striking given the simultaneous abstraction of the vector of contagion through the fundamentally mathematical language of electronic viruses. The advent of digital imaging technologies and the development of increasingly elaborate networks of electronic connectivity that can rapidly become chains of infection have resulted (once again) in a proliferation of representations of contagion. And the discursive intersections of global telecommunications and global contagion have exaggerated the sense of temporal as well as spatial reduction of distances between global outbreaks and local infestations, resulting in these most recent expressions of "penetration panic." As we saw in *The Silent Invader*, the visual embodiment of contagion has often been expressed through a collapse of disease and racial difference, conveyed through highly sexualized networks of infection. And yet, as the editors of a recent volume on race in digital representation have noted, "Race is rarely (if ever) as invisible offline as it is in cyberspace."[4] Similar observations have been made about the invisibility and consequent malleability of sexual identity online. In fact, Sherry Turkle links this invisibility to what she calls a widespread but "curiously irrational preoccupation" with "guessing the true gender of players behind MUD (Multi-User Domain) characters."[5] Nonetheless, cultural discourses surrounding the digital realm are heavily invested with racial and sexual imagery, as in the following interpretation of a technological virus in terms of human sexuality—an analysis that was repeated in countless commentaries on the Love Bug: "The extraordinary efficacy of the Love Bug was caused partly by its timing, striking as it did on a busy weekday morning, but also by its seductiveness. It was a minor masterpiece of what hackers like to call 'social engineering'—in other words, manipulating the rubes. Few of the lonely hearts among cubicle dwellers could resist its siren song."[6]

Here, the computer virus is a sexual predator, much like the widely noted "dirty old men" who pose as children in chat rooms, only to expose their innocent online victims to pornography or worse.[7] And the computer user's vulnerability to such malevolent seduction is based not on the simple fact that his or her work site is a networked computer but, rather, on a form of sexual "perversion" that actively seeks gratification through anonymous and disembodied sexual encounters. Thus, the "lonely hearts" who caught the virus (or, more precisely, whose computers caught the virus) are seen as both victims *and* perpetrators of the deception inherent in a technology of representation that flagrantly disregards traditional oppositions between real and imaginary, authentic and simulation. The dissolution of such oppositions undermines the rigid definition of categories of identity such as race and sexuality, replacing essentialist notions of subjectivity with far more fluid conceptions of embodiment. And yet, online chat rooms have also been linked to real-life outbreaks of sexually transmitted diseases.[8]

Another effect of this dissolution of boundaries between the real and the imaginary is that the digital imaging technologies used to represent the electronically interconnected world can seamlessly integrate the indexical and the artificial, thus fulfilling the world health fantasy of visualizing invisible contagions in everyday life. Although the advent of digital imaging has been widely recognized as eroding an earlier faith in photographic realism, the ability to convincingly represent an invisible element of the profilmic scene might be viewed as a development that invests the artificial image with an indexical veracity that is even more "real" than an unvarnished image ever could be. The "crisis of referentiality" that undermines the boundaries between authenticity and simulation in the postphotographic era thus finds a special case in the problem of visually representing invisible contagion. Lev Manovich has concisely summarized this paradox: "The logic of the digital photograph is one of historical continuity and discontinuity. The digital image tears apart the net of semiotic codes, modes of display, and patterns of spectatorship in modern visual culture—and, at the same time, weaves this net even stronger. The digital image annihilates photography while solidifying, glorifying and immortalizing the photographic."[9] But if a microscopic virus is invisible to the naked eye, does its consequent failure to appear on celluloid make it any less infectious? On the biological level, the answer is obviously no, but Manovich's description of the "logic of the digital photograph" equally describes the logic of world health, wherein it is the act of visual representation that simultaneously establishes the indexical presence of contagion, and, through the act of identification, eliminates the potency of the threat of contamination.

The repeated failure of earlier public health films accurately to capture a profilmic image of contagion might thus seem to be resolved by the advent of digital imaging technologies. With their ability to produce a convincingly authentic—albeit entirely simulated—representation of the spread of disease, digital media could potentially allay the anxiety that had driven earlier attempts to visualize the invisible. But instead, we find that "new" and "old" media occupy equally anxious relationships to "the real."[10] Moreover, contemporary metaphors of contagion, epitomized by the notion of the computer "virus," continue to draw upon the racialized and sexualized linkage of disease and difference, frequently through the discourse of AIDS.

PERPETUAL CONTAGION

The linkage of disease and difference has a long history that predates the invention of motion pictures. But the institutional and representational intersections between the fields of public health and cinema together have formed unique modes of imagining and monitoring the development of the public sphere and its bodies, particularly in relation to global technologies of transportation and communication. While cinema provided a means of visually representing the temporal and spatial flow of invisible contagions, thus aligning certain geographic and demographic characteristics with contamination (the "Third World" with racially and sexually "marked" bodies, for example), the medium also became a metaphor for the flow of contagion itself. Public health films strived toward realism, with the aim of producing representational inoculations against disease. Yet this very realism was seen as a source of "moral contagion" by the film reformers of the 1930s, who were also dedicated to sanitizing the public sphere. But as the examples of science fiction and more recent contagion and conspiracy films have shown, the formalized separation of education and entertainment did not effectively eliminate from Hollywood films the preoccupation with visually imaging the invisible spread of contagion. And as critiques of early HIV and AIDS videos have argued, the collapse of racial and sexual difference with disease continues to structure the audiovisual discourse of world health.[11]

The period after World War Two thus represents a moment of discursive consolidation, linking early cinema's fascination with the realm of movement and objects previously invisible to the naked eye (such as squirming bacteria in a petri dish) with the rhetoric of contagious globalization that continues to inform imaginations of the technologically enhanced future (jet airplanes and the World Wide Web rapidly connecting the farthest reaches of the planet). While earlier attempts to visually represent invisible contagions met with limited success, digital manipulations of the profilmic image smoothly integrate the indexical and the artificial. And yet, as contemporary popular and scientific cultures attest, the simulation of contagion perpetually defers visual access to "the real." Instead, the trope of contagion endlessly reproduces itself through a paranoid fantasy of internalized surveillance and universal contamination. The impossibility of capturing an authentic representation of contagion blurs the boundaries between image and reality, producing an effect that mimics the original anxiety: an omnipresence of absent pathogens.

Notes

1. Consider, for example, the widespread avoidance of restaurants in San Francisco's Chinatown during the SARS outbreak, despite the fact that no cases had been confirmed anywhere within U.S. borders. "The SARS Epidemic: Economic Fallout; Market for Chinese-American Delicacy Plummets." *New York Times*, May 23, 2003, A8.

2. My use of the term "indexical" follows from the works of semiotician C. S. Peirce and film theorist André Bazin. The term is discussed at length in chapter 2, but for present purposes, the key point is that indexical signs bear a causal (or existential) relationship to the object that they represent, as in the case of smoke signifying the existence of fire. Thus, an indexical image of contagion would function as concrete evidence that a pathogen exists in a specific temporal and spatial locale, as when a thermometer indexically proves that a patient is running a fever.

3. For more on the *Science of Life* series, see Eberwein, *Sex Ed*; Pernick, "Sex Education Films, U.S. Government, 1920s"; and Pernick, *The Black Stork*.

4. *How Disease Is Spread* (1924).

5. On the commodification of screen bodies, especially through the Hollywood star system, see Dyer, *Stars*; DeCordova, *Picture Personalities*; and Gledhill, *Stardom*. On the commodification of the motion picture audience, see Gomery, *Shared Pleasures*.

6. The classic account of the cinematic fragmentation of the human body, and particularly the female body, is Mulvey, "Visual Pleasure and Narrative Cinema."

7. See Linda Williams's excellent discussion of Marx's commodity fetish and Freud's sexual fetish in *Hard Core*.

8. Ginzberg, *Women and the Work of Benevolence*.

9. Sekula, "The Body and the Archive." See also Gunning, "Tracing the Individual Body."

The similarity of this late-nineteenth-century discourse to contemporary practices of racial profiling is suggestive of the extent to which the discourse of racialized contagion continues to pervade u.s. culture.

10. From this highly narrativized representation of the ever-expanding sphere of contagion spread by the tubercular woman, the film sums up the offending behavior without offering any solution, turning instead to a qualitatively different scenario of contagion, where a preventive measure *is* recommended. The intertitle announces, "We have seen how disease is spread through carelessness. In our homes we can further protect ourselves by thoroughly cleansing all raw food before serving it," followed by a series of medium close-ups of a woman scrubbing vegetables in a sink and then proudly displaying them to the camera, neatly stacked on a tray. While this sequence shares with the prior sequence a preoccupation with the domestic sphere of consumption, there is no attempt to produce a coherent diegesis, and just as abruptly as the focus jumped from the spread of tuberculosis to food preparation, the next intertitle raises another problem: "Tuberculosis, 'flu,' pneumonia, and common colds may be disseminated in a fine spray discharged by coughing or sneezing." This unrelated announcement is followed by a scene in which two girls are playing checkers and a boy sits by, watching. One of the girls sneezes, and the next intertitle explains that she should always cover her nose and mouth with her own handkerchief. In the next scene, the girl sneezes again, but follows the proper disease-prevention protocol, and the film unexpectedly comes to an end.

11. On advertising and the culture of consumption in the early twentieth century, see Marchand, *Advertising the American Dream*; Fox and Lears, *The Culture of Consumption*. See also Tomes, *The Gospel of Germs*, for a discussion of the advertisement of hygiene products.

12. Peiss, *Cheap Amusements*; Rabinovitz, *For the Love of Pleasure*; S. Ewen, *Captains of Consciousness*; and Ewen and Ewen, *Channels of Desire*.

13. This concept was developed in B. Anderson, *Imagined Communities*.

14. While films such as the *Science of Life* series may have shown frequently in noncommercial venues, no systematic regulation of the types of films shown in public theaters took place until the Production Code was revised in 1934. On the discourse of "separate spheres" and objections to women leaving the private sphere for the public, see Smith-Rosenberg, *Disorderly Conduct*; and Scott, *Gender and the Politics of History*.

15. My argument that the discourse of globalization only enters these film genres (and popular culture in general) *after* World War Two is not meant to imply that the American motion picture industry only became "global" in the postwar period. On the contrary, the discursive globalization that I identify lags far behind the economic globalization of cinema. For a thoroughly documented argument that Hollywood was already a global culture industry long before World War Two, see Thompson, *Exporting Entertainment*.

16. For an excellent discussion of the dominant modes of visual representation in early-twentieth-century medicine, see Cartwright, *Screening the Body*. Most of the films Cartwright discusses are primarily scientific and not directed toward a general audience, with the major exception of her discussion of postwar tuberculosis films.

17. The only productions sponsored by federal government agencies between the wars were the non-health-related films of the short-lived U.S. Film Service—a New Deal program that funded the celebrated social realist films of Pare Lorentz, *The Plow That Broke the Plains* (1936) and *The River* (1938). See Snyder, *Pare Lorentz and the Documentary Film.* For a complete history of the U.S. Film Service and other interwar federal filmmaking, see MacCann, *The People's Films.*

18. In fact, very little scholarship on public health film exists. The important works are cited in later chapters, but here I wish to call attention to a special issue of *American Literary History* on contagion and culture, edited by Wald, Tomes, and Lynch, that does not address film per se but is nonetheless useful in its thematic linkage.

19. For a thorough and extremely useful discussion of the challenges of researching ephemeral films, see the introduction in Schaefer, *"Bold! Daring! Shocking! True!"*

20. For a more extensive critique of film analysis based on the director's intentions, see Caughie, *Theories of Authorship.*

21. For a thorough discussion of the use value and pitfalls of ethnographic evidence, see Staiger, *Interpreting Films.*

22. Vasey, *The World According to Hollywood.*

1 PUBLIC SPHERE AS PETRI DISH

1. Apart from the occasional documentary that makes it to mainstream exhibition, the commingling of documentary and fiction films tends to occur only in commercially marginal art-house theaters.

2. The prominent status of *Panic in the Streets* within the discourse of public health was evidenced by a display at the National Library of Medicine (on the campus of the National Institutes of Health in Bethesda, Maryland) in 1998, commemorating the 100-year anniversary of the United States Public Health Service (USPHS) by displaying promotional posters and other materials depicting the film.

3. See Kraut, *Silent Travelers.* Consistent with the public responses to the outbreaks of yellow fever and cholera in the nineteenth century, which blamed the former on German immigrants and the latter on Irish newcomers, the first highly politicized public health case of the twentieth century in the United States centered on fears of racial contamination in the outbreak of bubonic plague in San Francisco's Chinatown in 1900. For more on this case, see Mullan, *Plagues and Politics*; and Shah, *Contagious Divides.*

4. The linkage of rats and ethnic others has a long history in various racist traditions, notably in anti-Semitic imagery. See *The Architecture of Doom* (1989), a documentary on the construction of a fascist style in the public spaces of Nazi Germany, for several clips from animated Nazi propaganda films that display this particular racist visual construction of disease and difference.

5. Reports of typhus fever epidemics in Europe prompted the USPHS to expand surveillance practices by placing their own inspectors in overseas ports, supervising the examinations of intended U.S. immigrants by local physicians. The systematic pursuit of invisible

germs brought steamship companies under surveillance as well; they were "required to establish bathing and disinfection facilities to insure the delousing of passengers from infected areas. Service officers supervised such procedures and made terminal inspections as a prerequisite to issuance of bills of health." If a government or a steamship were noncompliant with the Public Health Service, the ships would be penalized upon arrival in the United States—they would be held in quarantine and fined. R.C. Williams, *The United States Public Health Service*, 88.

6. The National Health Council, an association for national voluntary health organizations, was founded in 1921 to coordinate services for its constituent members, including mounting its own campaigns against disease. An important activity of the council was the distribution of health publications, such as health film and poster lists, as well as distribution of the films themselves. Means, *A History of Health Education in the United States*, 177. Similarly, the National Tuberculosis Association established a Health Education Service in 1928, under the direction of Dr. H. E. Kleinschmidt, an active promoter of the use of cinema for health education. Ibid., 187. Kleinschmidt's work is discussed extensively in Eberwein, *Sex Ed*, and in the Adolf Nichtenhauser papers at the National Library of Medicine, which Eberwein draws upon extensively in his own discussion. The American Public Health Association also created a Health Education Section in 1922, and numerous commercial companies, such as the Metropolitan Life Insurance Company, became involved in health education through film production during the 1920s, "as a secondary function to supplement their major purpose of selling a particular product." Means, *A History of Health Education in the United States*, 216.

7. The subsequent sequestering of health films into educational exhibition contexts should not be viewed as evidence of the films' discursive marginality; on the contrary, the techniques for visualizing invisible contagions in postwar public health films permeated mass culture as well, particularly the newly popular genre of science fiction. Some notable exceptions to the government monopoly on health film production were the *Encyclopedia Britannica*'s and the Metropolitan Insurance Company's series of health and safety films. Most of the nongovernmental producers of health films in this period used the films as advertising media.

8. A notable exception, both prior to and after the Production Code was revised in 1934, was the production of pseudo-educational exploitation films, such as sex films that were ostensibly instructing their audiences in methods for avoiding venereal diseases, and mental hygiene films like *Reefer Madness* (1938). Robert Eberwein cites the following sex education films that were produced by commercial—not government—agencies between the *Science of Life* series and World War Two: *The Reproductive System* (1924–27?); *Are You Fit to Marry?* (1927); *The Naked Truth* (1927); *Pitfalls of Passion* (1927); *The Venereal Diseases* (1928); *Miracle of Birth* (1930s); *Damaged Lives* (1933); *What Price Innocence* (1933); *Guilty Parents* (1934); *High School Girl* (1934); *Modern Motherhood* (1934); *Birth of a Baby* (1937); *Damaged Goods* (1937); *Human Wreckage* (1938). Eberwein, *Sex Ed*, 235–41.

9. Duffy, *The Sanitarians*, 216.

10. As Means and others have demonstrated, films were not widely seen as legitimate or necessary educational expenditures until after their instructional and propagandistic effects were clearly proven during World War Two. See Means, *A History of Health Education in the United States*; Essex-Lopresti, "The Medical Film 1897–1997, Part I"; and Smith, *Mental Hygiene*. For an excellent discussion of the use of film and other audiovisual media in the classroom, see Goldfarb, *Visual Pedagogy*. As Martin Pernick has documented, *The Science of Life* series was "begun during the war but first released in 1922, [and] these films were distributed officially for the next fifteen years and remained in use by some school boards and health departments for many decades afterward." "Sex Education," 766.

11. On immigration and the Progressive reform movement, see E. Ewen, *Immigrant Women in the Land of Dollars*; Peiss, *Cheap Amusements*; and Wiebe, *The Search for Order*.

12. On the early history and discourses of cinema censorship, see Jowett, *Film*; Kuhn, *Cinema, Censorship and Sexuality*; and Lea Jacobs, *The Wages of Sin*.

13. For an example of the use and production of films in the settlement house movement, see Addams, *The Spirit of Youth and the City Streets*. See also Sloan, *The Loud Silents*.

14. Huettig, *Economic Control of the Motion Picture Industry*, 45.

15. Eventually the film's earnings topped $3.5 million. D. Cook, *A History of Narrative Film*, 246.

16. Lewis Jacobs, *The Rise of the American Film*, 419–32. See also Doherty, *Pre-Code Hollywood*; and Smulyan, *Selling Radio*.

17. The exoticism of the nonwhite body and its linkage with disease are also collapsed in later Hollywood films. For an excellent discussion of the temporal and spatial boundary between premodern and modern bodies, see Rony, "*King Kong* and the Monster in Ethnographic Cinema," in *The Third Eye*.

18. Paul W. Facey, historian of the Catholic Legion of Decency, assessed the development of the talkies as follows: "As the movies matured, in content and in technique, the cruder violations of the standards of sex behavior gave way to the more subtle. The coming of talking pictures accentuated the trend, opening the door, through dialogue, to a wider horizon of ideas than could be conveyed by the pantomime of the silent films. . . . Talking pictures, keeping the visual elements of the earlier pictures, had added a greater degree of sophistication, and there appeared a greater emphasis upon objection to the immorality of the ideas which it was claimed the movies were inculcating into their patrons. The charge that 'evil is made to appear good' became the feature objection." Facey, *The Legion of Decency*, 8–9.

19. Doherty, *Pre-Code Hollywood*, 5–6.

20. Historian John Duffy has noted the centrality of communication systems in establishing a nationwide network of public health departments in the 1930s, especially after the Social Security Act of 1935 greatly expanded state health departments. Duffy, *The Sanitarians*, 218, 258.

21. In 1964, Potter Stewart, Associate Justice of the U.S. Supreme Court, immortalized this formulation in his opinion on pornography: "I shall not today attempt further to define the kinds of material . . . but I know it when I see it." Simpson, *Simpson's Contemporary Quotations.*

22. G. Black, *Hollywood Censored*, 169–70; and Lea Jacobs, *The Wages of Sin*, 21–22.

23. G. Black, *Hollywood Censored*, 171.

24. Ibid.

25. Ibid.

26. Ibid., 171–72. And the Supreme Court agreed with them—motion pictures were not protected by the First Amendment until 1952. See Jowett, "'A Significant Medium for the Communication of Ideas.'"

27. G. Black, *Hollywood Censored*, 172.

28. From the text of "The Production Code of the Motion Picture Producers and Directors of America, Inc.," reprinted in Jowett, *Film*, 468.

29. Huettig, *Economic Control of the Motion Picture Industry*, 116; Couvares, "Hollywood, Main Street, and the Church," 596.

30. Jowett, Jarvie, and Fuller, *Children and the Movies*, 28.

31. Jowett, *Film*, 176–77 and 465–67. See the appendices in *Film* for the complete texts of Hollywood's early attempts at self-regulation.

32. As early as 1926, a group of motion picture reformers marched on Washington, D.C., demanding federal regulation of the movies. Leading the charge were Reverend William H. Short, who would soon become executive director of the Motion Picture Research Council, and Canon William Sheafe Chase, director of the Federal Motion Picture Council in America, along with over two hundred representatives of women's organizations. Recognizing that reform efforts aimed at federal censorship of motion pictures had failed because of a lack of scientific evidence to support their claims, Reverend Short obtained funding for the Payne Fund Studies in 1928, under the auspices of the Motion Picture Research Council. G. Black, "Hollywood Censored," 170. Jowett, Jarvie, and Fuller, *Children and the Movies*, 2, 27.

33. This theory of film spectatorship, often described as the "hypodermic needle" model, gained great currency in the 1930s and continues to circulate widely in popular reports on the deleterious effects of mass media on youth. While this theory correctly recognizes the important ideological function of technologies of mass entertainment, it fails to acknowledge the material conditions of existence that precede (and surround) the encounter with cinema. The conventionalized rhetoric of "injection" is particularly suggestive when considered in the context of the film reform debates that construed spectatorship as an occasion for moral and physical contagion. Within this rhetoric, gangster movies—rather than economic desperation and other complex causes—are blamed for high crime rates and violence in poor urban neighborhoods. The industry's commonly cited defense, that motion pictures simply "reflect" the society and historical period in which they are produced, ac-

knowledges the unavoidable historicity of all cultural productions but fails to account for the complex range of factors that can overdetermine the relationship between a cultural product and its production and reception contexts.

34. The Payne Fund Studies, all published by Macmillan in New York, were Charters, *Motion Pictures and Youth*; Holaday, *Getting Ideas From the Movies*; Peterson and Thurstone, *Motion Pictures and the Social Attitudes of Children*; Shuttleworth and May, *The Social Conduct and Attitudes of Movie Fans*; Dysinger and Ruckmick, *The Emotional Responses of Children to the Motion Picture Situation*; Peters, *Motion Pictures and Standards of Morality*; Renshaw, *Children's Sleep*; Blumer, *Movies and Conduct*; Dale, *The Content of Motion Pictures, Children's Attendance at Motion Pictures*, and *How to Appreciate Motion Pictures*; Blumer and Hauser, *Movies, Delinquency, and Crime*. Paul G. Cressey's and Frederick M. Thrasher's intended report, "Boys, Movies, and City Streets," cited in the list of studies titled "Motion Pictures and Youth: The Payne Fund Studies" in the frontispiece of each volume published by Macmillan, 1933–35, was not completed. The summary of the studies was Forman, *Our Movie Made Children*. The Motion Picture Research Council's support for government regulation of block booking indicates the group's stance in decided opposition to self-regulation by the film industry and in favor of prior censorship by the federal government. This, in turn, strongly suggests that Short intended in advance to use the ostensibly objective scientific investigations in a campaign against the film industry. With the studios already on the defensive, Short arranged, with Werrett Wallace Charters (director of the studies), to have Henry James Forman publish *Our Movie Made Children*—a sensationalized layperson's summary of the findings—in 1933, in advance of the studies themselves. Lea Jacobs, "Reformers and Spectators," 31–32. Excerpts of Forman's book were also published as articles in popular magazines, including *McCall's*. Jowett, Jarvie, and Fuller, *Children and the Movies*, 7.

35. Around the same time that the studies were being conducted, Mortimer Adler, a professor of philosophy and law at the University of Chicago, was pursuing his own investigation into the morals and politics of motion pictures, published as *Art and Prudence: A Study in Practical Philosophy*. While the Payne Fund Studies tended toward a behaviorist approach to film spectatorship, Adler's volume challenged the very presumption that motion pictures have any necessary "effect" on their viewers at all. As with the scientific language of the Payne Fund Studies, Adler's philosophical treatise required translation for dissemination to the general public, so a brief summary of his work was written by Raymond Moley and published in 1938, "at the suggestion of representatives of the motion picture industry," under a title that emphasized its opposition to the Payne Fund summary: *Are We Movie-Made?* (viii). These "representatives of the motion picture industry" probably included Will Hays, then president of the Motion Picture Producers and Distributors of America (MPPDA). Moley had done some writing for Hays during his earlier career in the Republican National Party and was also the author of the only official history of the MPPDA at that time, *The Hays Office*. Adler, too, was encouraged by the motion picture industry

to dedicate a section of his book to an in-depth critique of the Payne Fund Studies. As noted in the preface to *Art and Prudence*, "As a result of their reading [Adler's earlier work] *Crime, Law and Social Science*, representatives of the motion picture producers asked me to review for them the recent empirical investigations specifically concerned with the influence of motion pictures on human behavior." Adler became a paid consultant to the MPPDA around the time Moley's book was published. Adler, *Art and Prudence*, xi; and Jowett, Jarvie, and Fuller, *Children and the Movies*, xx, 116–17, 366n93. Author Raymond Moley sarcastically described the popularity of *Our Movie Made Children* in the preface to his own book, noting that the misguided public embrace of Forman's book demanded that its fallacious claims be rebutted. Moley summarizes Adler's debunking of the Payne Fund Studies as "a challenging demonstration of the dangers inherent in the incompetent use of scientific methods in the field of the social sciences. It refutes, word by word, a series of pretentious attempts to 'prove' that the motion picture causes delinquency and crime, or has other corrupting influences on character and conduct. The sharp edge of analytic reason moves through the half-truths and prejudicial conclusions of these studies like a keen scythe in a clump of weeds." Moley, *Are We Movie-Made?* vi, 18. Unfortunately, it was too late—the revised Production Code had gone into effect in 1934, and it would govern the content of the world's largest and most culturally influential output of motion pictures for the next several decades.

36. As the ensuing attempts to answer this same question have demonstrated, social scientific attempts to specify the effects of film viewing have produced contradictory results at best. The current debates over the effects of violent movies and television clearly demonstrate the continued difficulty of proving that motion pictures cause violent behavior in their viewers. Nonetheless, the studies continue, and, in their time, the Payne Fund Studies did achieve a new level of systematicity in their pursuit of scientific objectivity. For summary histories of social science research on mass communications, see Delia, "Communication Research"; and Jowett, Reath, and Schouten, "The Control of Mass Entertainment Media in Canada, the United States and Great Britain."

37. The only book-length study of the Payne Fund Studies, a self-described "reclamation" of the studies, is Jowett, Jarvie, and Fuller, *Children and the Movies*. Other discussions of the Payne Fund Studies from the perspective of mass communications include Fearing, "Influence of Movies on Attitudes and Behavior"; Handel, *Hollywood Looks at Its Audience*; and Lowery and De Fleur, *Milestones in Mass Communications Research*. From the perspective of film studies, the Payne Fund Studies are briefly mentioned in another volume whose title reflects, if indirectly, the language of the Payne Fund: Sklar, *Movie-Made America*. See also Jowett, *Film*; G. Black, *Hollywood Censored*, 150–55; and Balio, *Grand Design*, 3, 56. In a recent collection of essays (Bernstein, *Controlling Hollywood*) the Payne Fund Studies only appear twice, though they are attributed a central role in forcing the Production Code Administration (PCA) to intensify the enforcement of its rulings starting in 1934 and for setting the terms of the censorship discourse for the next two decades. See Vasey, "Beyond Sex and Violence"; and Draper, "'Controversy Has Probably Destroyed Forever the Context.'"

38. M. Anderson, *The Modern Goliath*; and Perlman, *The Movies on Trial*. For a brief discussion of these texts, see Draper, " 'Controversy Has Probably Destroyed Forever the Context.' "

39. A brief selection of representative titles includes Hoban, *Movies That Teach*; Fern, *Teaching with Films*; Gipson, *Films in Business and Industry*; Gibson, *Motion Picture Testing and Research*; Elliott, *Film and Education*; Nelson, *Mass Media and Education*; Film Evaluation Board of the Advisory Board on Education and Division of Mathematics, *The Use of Films and Television in Mathematics Education*; May and Lumsdaine, *Learning from Films*.

40. As Ruth Vasey has argued, "The [Payne Fund] studies arguably constituted the single most influential factor in the decision to publicly restructure and strengthen the office of the PCA in 1934." Vasey, "Beyond Sex and Violence," 127n42. See also Lea Jacobs, *The Wages of Sin*, 19; and Doherty, *Pre-Code Hollywood*, 320.

41. Forman, *Our Movie Made Children*, 6.

42. Legion of Decency, *Motion Pictures Classified by National Legion of Decency*.

43. Forman, *Our Movie Made Children*, 25–28.

44. While Forman's *Our Movie Made Children* is the primary text under analysis here, the language used in that volume is culled from the Payne Fund Studies themselves, which are, in turn, responding to the reform discourses of the period. My citation of Forman as representative of a broader discourse, therefore, should not be taken as attributing agency to Forman as sole or original "author" of these ideas about the relationship between motion pictures, education, and public health.

45. Jowett, Jarvie, and Fuller, *Children and the Movies*, 362n45.

46. Forman, *Our Movie Made Children*, 63.

47. Ibid., 121.

48. Ibid., 98.

49. Blumer and Hauser, *Movies, Delinquency, and Crime*, 46–47. See also Forman, *Our Movie Made Children*, 113.

50. Forman, *Our Movie Made Children*, 274, 2–3.

51. Ibid., 66–67.

52. Perhaps it would be more accurate to say that the reformers were attempting to convert "nonwhite" immigrants into "white" citizens. The boundaries between categories of race and ethnicity were often quite blurry and malleable in this period. See Omi and Winant, *Racial Formation in the United States*; Dyer, *White*; Roediger, *The Wages of Whiteness*; Jacobson, *Whiteness of a Different Color*; Hill, *Whiteness*. For a discussion of this topic that specifically addresses the cinema, see Bernardi, *The Birth of Whiteness*.

53. Jowett, Jarvie, and Fuller, *Children and the Movies*, 66–74. Paul Facey confirms the pro-federal censorship stance of the Motion Picture Research Council in *The Legion of Decency*, 186.

54. Jowett, Jarvie, and Fuller, *Children and the Movies*, 362–63n45.

55. Forman, *Our Movie Made Children*, 232.

56. Ibid., 88. Emphasis in original.

57. Ibid., 68.

58. Ibid., 237.

59. Facey, *The Legion of Decency*, 112.

60. Ibid., 114.

61. Legion of Decency, *Motion Pictures Classified by National Legion of Decency*, 84. *Mom and Dad* was an uncredited remake of a 1934 film, *High School Girl*, but it also recycled some segments from the 1942 Navy training film, *Sex Hygiene*, and from the 1941 USPHS film, *In Defense of the Nation*. See Schaefer, *"Bold! Daring! Shocking! True!"*; Eberwein, *Sex Ed*; and White, *"Mom and Dad* (1944)."

62. Jowett, *Film*, 468–72.

63. Pernick, *The Black Stork*, 121–24. *The Black Stork*, a eugenicist euthanasia film made in 1917, is extensively discussed in Pernick's eponymously titled book.

64. G. Black, "Hollywood Censored," 178.

65. Ibid. Here, Black is citing "Compensating Moral Values," June 13, 1934, box 47, Will Hays Papers, Indiana State Historical Society, Indianapolis.

66. Vasey, *The World According to Hollywood*, 100–101.

67. Ibid., 101.

68. P. Rosen, "Document and Documentary," 64. For more on Grierson, see Barnouw, *Documentary*.

69. P. Rosen, "Document and Documentary," 66.

70. Ibid., 67.

2 "NONINFECTED BUT INFECTIBLE"

1. For a discussion of the importance of border crossing to debates about postmodern hybridity and postwar globalization, see Jameson, *Postmodernism, or, The Cultural Logic of Late Capitalism*. See also Joyrich, *Re-Viewing Reception*.

2. On the anxious production of coherent subjectivity through postwar Hollywood film, see Silverman, "Historical Trauma and Male Subjectivity."

3. Following from semiotician C. S. Peirce's distinction between iconic, indexical, and symbolic signs, I am invoking the category of the indexical to indicate a type of semiotic sign that is in a causal or existential relation to the object it represents. The classic examples of indexical signs are a weathercock, a barometer, or smoke signifying the existence of fire. The causal relationship is what distinguishes an indexical sign from an iconic sign, which functions through similarity or resemblance to the object it represents (as in a portrait or a diagram), and from a symbolic sign, which functions through convention, as in the case of language where the word "cat" refers to an animal that we recognize by that name for purely arbitrary reasons. In the case of photographic or cinematic signs, the image is iconic in that it functions through resemblance, but it is indexical in that it contains what Bazin would call an "ontological" link between the profilmic event and the photographic representation.

The key distinction here is between photographic images that claim to have an indexical or unmediated relationship to "the real," as in the case of documentary films of this period, and images that bear no necessary relationship to reality but claim that they do. This is not to imply that there *are* forms of representation that have an unmediated relationship to reality, but rather that some representational forms *claim* that they directly represent "the real," even if they do not. For a discussion of the significance of Peirce's theory of indexicality to the field of cinema studies, see Stam, Burgoyne, and Flitterman-Lewis, *New Vocabularies in Film Semiotics*.

4. It is important to note that this oscillation usually takes place within a single film; that is, *both* the indexical *and* the artificial poles are mobilized in most of the films under investigation here.

5. In a sense, then, the public health films produced in this period fit in with the "New Deal" style of documentary filmmaking described by Paul Arthur in "Jargons of Authenticity (Three American Moments)," but these films simultaneously invoke the mode of constituting cinematic authority typical of the dominant style of the period and presume a cinema verité epistemological stance, based on their faith in the truth of "unmediated" images and sounds. For more on these distinctions, see Arthur, "Jargons of Authenticity (Three American Moments)."

6. Bazin, *What Is Cinema?* 14. Bazin goes on to argue that "every image is to be seen as an object and every object as an image" (ibid., 16). This is not to elide Bazin's own privileging of deep focus cinematography, which "reintroduced ambiguity into the structure of the image" (ibid., 36)—space does not permit an extended discussion of the distinctions between Bazin's emphasis on the indexicality of the image and his praise of the potential ambiguity of cinematic representation—suffice it to say that the public health films under discussion here would fall within Bazin's category of films that "put their faith in reality" and therefore, maintain their indexical qualities.

7. Gunning, "An Aesthetic of Astonishment."

8. The concept of "aesthetic censorship" comes from Pernick, *The Black Stork*, 123.

9. The key distinction here is between cinematic images and sounds that issue from a preexisting profilmic time and space, and thus constitute a manipulated but nonetheless documentary "chunk of reality," and images and sounds (animation and voiceover, respectively) that are created in postproduction, and thus bear a more obviously mediated, "nondocumentary" relation to the objects they represent. Although these strategies would seem to occupy opposing positions in relation to "realism," they both nonetheless claim privileged access to "the real."

10. For an excellent analysis of the early medical and scientific uses of cinema, see Cartwright, *Screening the Body*. On the intersection of medicine and more contemporary moving images, see Treichler, Cartwright, and Penley, *The Visible Woman*.

11. Kraut, *Silent Travelers*, 30. Kraut's text is the definitive analysis of the linkage of disease and difference in the history of immigration to the United States.

12. Duffy, *The Sanitarians*, 193.

13. See ibid., 179, for a discussion of the ongoing linkage of recent immigrants' bodies with disease in late-nineteenth-century popular media, despite the low incidence of the diseases being discursively invoked.

14. One of the earliest films to use animation in the pursuit of science—albeit the comedic pursuit of science—was *Les Joyeux Microbes* (1909).

15. On the Spanish American War and early cinema, see Musser, *Before the Nickelodeon*, especially 126–33; and Castonguay, "The Spanish American War in u.s. Media Culture." See also Musser, *The Emergence of Cinema*; and Fell, *Film Before Griffith*.

16. R. C. Williams, *The United States Public Health Service*, 86–87.

17. See Elsaesser, *Early Cinema*; Doane, "Temporality, Storage, Legibility"; Braun, *Picturing Time*.

18. For an analysis of the status of the female body in these investigations, see L. Williams, "Film Body." On the racial uses of early scientific cinema, especially ethnographic documentary, see Rony, *The Third Eye*.

19. Among the public health films to be discussed in this book, the "microscopic" animation of contagion can be found in *The Science of Life* (1924); *Tsutsugamushi* (1945); *Fight Syphilis* (1941); *Know for Sure* (1941); *To the People of the United States* (1944); *They Do Come Back* (1940); and *Hospital Sepsis* (1959). As demonstrated in *Hemolytic Streptococcus Control* (1945) and *The Eternal Fight* (1948), rudimentary animation techniques gained a popularity comparable to that enjoyed by microscopic images (and later, by X-ray images). In fact, numerous public health films would eventually replace microscopic images with stop-action insertions of visible signifiers of germs, such as little black stars at the site of contagion, as in *How Disease Is Spread* (1924). It is thus quite significant that Bray Studios, the production company that coproduced the first u.s. Public Health Service health films, was a pioneer in animation techniques.

20. Gunning, "The Cinema of Attractions."

21. Cartwright, *Screening the Body*, xiii.

22. Pernick, *The Black Stork*, 119.

23. Furman, *A Profile of the United States Public Health Service*, 312. The production company responsible for the "Safety First" films is unknown. See also the discussions of traveling health education in the 1910 Louisiana health train, which also employed motion pictures, in Means, *A History of Health Education in the United States*, 77–109; and Duffy, *The Sanitarians*, 227. On the intersecting histories of the railroad and motion pictures, see Kirby, *Parallel Tracks*.

24. Duffy, *The Sanitarians*, 242–43.

25. The clearest examples of such assessments are the linkage of strong troops in World War One with anti–venereal disease campaigns; Nazi Germany's obsession with eugenics, physical fitness, and social hygiene; and later, the endless Cold War comparisons of the physical and mental health of American and Soviet youths.

26. For statistics on immigration, see Kraut, *Silent Travelers*. See also Hoerder, *Cultures in Contact*; Dinnerstein and Reimers, *Ethnic Americans*; Gabaccia, *Immigration and American Diversity*.

27. R. C. Williams, *The United States Public Health Service*, 101–11.

28. Means, *A History of Health Education in the United States*, 112–13.

29. *Fit to Fight* has been discussed extensively elsewhere: for a discussion of this film in the context of the history of sex education films, see Eberwein, *Sex Ed*, especially chapter 1, "The Initial Phase, 1914–1939," 15–62. See also Parascondola, "VD at the Movies"; and Pernick, *The Black Stork*. On the *Fit to Fight* campaign, see R. C. Williams, *The United States Public Health Service*, 592. The film's title was changed to *Fit to Win* for continued exhibition after the war ended. Thanks to Martin Pernick for bringing to my attention the copy of *Fit to Fight* held at the University of Michigan Historical Health Film Collection.

30. MacCann, *The People's Films*, 44–46. In addition to their educational function in the military campaign against venereal diseases, motion pictures were employed to promote patriotism and rally public support for U.S. involvement in World War One. To this end, President Wilson appointed the Committee on Public Information (the Creel Committee), which commissioned artists to make war posters, and also enlisted 75,000 Four Minute Men to speak daily in motion picture theaters and schoolhouses across the country to promote the war. Furman, *A Profile of the United States Public Health Service*, 316–17. See also Mock and Larson, *Words That Won the War*.

31. Moving images of combat were also collected by the army's Signal Corps and edited for the public by the Creel Committee, as well as being distributed for use in newsreels and other army training films. For a history of official federal filmmaking activities that does *not* address public health films, see MacCann, *The People's Films*. See also R. Wood, *Film and Propaganda in America*; Isenberg, *War on Film*; Dibbets and Hogenkamp, *Film and the First World War*; Mould, *American Newsfilm*; DeBauche, *Reel Patriotism*; Ward, *The Motion Picture Goes to War*; Campbell, *Reel America and World War I*.

32. Furman, *A Profile of the United States Public Health Service*, 360; and R. C. Williams, *The United States Public Health Service*, 93.

33. Furman, *A Profile of the United States Public Health Service*, 373–74.

34. R. C. Williams, *The United States Public Health Service*, 93.

35. As JoAnne Brown has argued in a discussion of the linkage of "modern conveniences" with invisible germs in early-twentieth-century advertising, "The telephone, with its close proximity to the mouth and ear and its conveyance of the invisible across a great distance, was a particular concern." Brown, "Crime, Commerce, and Contagionism," 68.

36. The gap between image and sound in this film is similar to the gap between story and discourse theorized by Emile Benveniste in *Problems in General Linguistics* and taken up in film and television studies by Margaret Morse in "The Television News Personality and Credibility."

37. A suggestively similar dynamic informs the relationship between vision and "the

real" in *Invasion of the Body Snatchers* (1956). The central protagonist of that film is also a medical doctor who fails to interpret the signs of difference as signs of alien invasion.

38. On the naval collapse of homosociality and homosexuality, see Chauncey, "Christian Brotherhood or Sexual Perversion?"

39. Put simply, there is no gender equivalent to the category of "sexually transmitted disease," and it is this difference that is highlighted through a comparison of *How Disease Is Spread* with the postwar films.

40. Foucault, *The History of Sexuality, Volume I*, 70.

41. On the role of the railroad in discourses of modernity that were engaged with the threat of the unknown masses in the public sphere, see Schivelbusch, *The Railway Journey*. See also Kirby, *Parallel Tracks*.

42. As McClintock explains, "According to the colonial version of this trope, imperial progress across the space of empire is figured as a journey backward in time to an anachronistic moment of prehistory. . . . Geographical difference across *space* is figured as a historical difference across *time*." McClintock, *Imperial Leather*, 40.

43. Given the post–World War Two context, one wonders whether this "X" is meant to represent the nuclear annihilation that finally ended the war. The discursive slippage between eliminating disease and eliminating the source of disease reappears in some later Hollywood films, such as *The Andromeda Strain* (1971), *The Crazies* (1973), and *Outbreak* (1995); in each of these films, the option of dropping a nuclear bomb on the infected area is seriously considered as the only solution that will halt the universal spread of disease.

44. As Mary Ann Doane has argued, "Despite a number of experiments with other types of sound/image relationships . . . synchronous dialogue remains the dominant form of sonorous representation in the cinema." Doane, "The Voice in the Cinema," 336.

45. The strategies by which the classical Hollywood cinema constructs an apparent unity of images and sounds are extensively analyzed in Bordwell and Thompson, *Film Art*.

46. On countercinematic oppositions to Hollywood form and style, see Comolli and Narboni, "Cinema/Ideology/Criticism" and "Parenthesis or Indirect Route"; MacCabe, "Realism and the Cinema"; Willemen, "The Third Cinema Question" and other essays in *Questions of Third Cinema*, edited by Pines and Willemen.

47. On the global economic dominance of the Hollywood film industry, see Balio, *Hollywood in the Age of Television*.

48. Doane, "The Voice in the Cinema," 335–36.

3 FROM INNER TO OUTER SPACE

1. Puar and Rai, "Monster, Terrorist, Fag."

2. Duffy, *The Sanitarians*, 269–73.

3. As Means and others have demonstrated, audiovisual aids were used extensively in public schools and other commercial and institutional settings only *after* World War Two. See Means, *A History of Health Education in the United States*; Essex-Lopresti, "The Medical Film 1897–1997, Part I"; Smith, *Mental Hygiene*.

4. Duffy, *The Sanitarians*, 279. As John Duffy, a historian of medicine, has noted, the end of World War Two brought more than economic prosperity and global hegemony to the United States; the period also saw major developments in medicine and surgery, both greatly assisted by advances in bacteriology that led to the discovery of penicillin. With such apparent progress occurring on all fronts, postwar confidence in the triumph of science and technology reached unprecedented heights, most clearly exemplified by the equally unparalleled federal and private funding available for medical research in this period. The National Institutes of Health (a separate institution of the USPHS) expanded at the same time the Centers for Disease Control did, as a result of substantially increased federal support of biomedical research in the postwar period. See also G. Rosen, *A History of Public Health*.

5. For an elaboration of this approach see the work of Bruno Latour, especially *Science in Action*.

6. The concept of a "social imaginary" is borrowed from Elsaesser, "Primary Identification and the Historical Subject."

7. I am not arguing that one set of metaphors simply stands in for another, but rather that they are interwoven. For a discussion of illness in general, and AIDS in particular, as a category that is filled with various metaphoric meanings that change frequently throughout history, see Sontag, *Illness as Metaphor and AIDS and Its Metaphors*.

8. The rise of image culture is perhaps most notably indicated by the publication, popularity, and enduring influence of three texts that emerged from the postwar period: Boorstin's *The Image, or What Happened to the American Dream* in 1961, McLuhan's "The Medium Is the Message" in *Understanding Media* in 1964, and Debord's *The Society of the Spectacle* in 1967.

9. Tarratt, "Monsters from the Id," 348. *Destination Moon* (1950). While *Destination Moon* is usually cited (often with *Rocketship X-M*, also released in 1950) as establishing science fiction film as a *coherent* genre, it should be noted that films representing fantastical scenarios, including extraterrestrial travel, are as old as the medium of film itself. See for instance the 1902 Georges Méliès film, *Le voyage dans la lune* (*A Trip to the Moon*). A useful source on the historical development of the science fiction film genre is Hardy, *Science Fiction*.

10. For a discussion of the use of stock footage in exploitation films, see Schaefer, "*Bold! Daring! Shocking! True!*" especially chapter 2, "'A Hodge-Podge of Cuttings and Splicings.' The Mode of Production and the Style of Classical Exploitation Films." See also McCarthy and Flynn, *Kings of the B's*. Even the popular horror and science fiction novelist Stephen King has commented that "the fears expressed [in horror films] are sociopolitical in nature, a fact that gives . . . Don Siegel's *Invasion of the Body Snatchers* . . . a crazily convincing documentary feel." King, "Danse Macabre," 1989.

11. Ironically, considering its celebrated "realism," *Destination Moon* won an Academy Award for Special Effects in 1950. Hardy, *Science Fiction*, 125.

12. For an excellent discussion of the "film within the film" (or *mise en abyme*) technique

in sex education films, see Eberwein, *Sex Ed*, especially chapter 2, "World War II and the Attack on Venereal Disease."

13. On the cover of the newspaper that tops the pile is the headline "United Nations Assembly Meets, Votes for Peace." As I discuss below, the United Nations attains iconographic prominence in science fiction films of the 1950s.

14. Knee, *The American Science Fiction Film and Fifties Culture*, 74–75.

15. Sontag, *Against Interpretation, and Other Essays*. 210.

16. *Them!* (1954).

17. *The War of the Worlds* (1953).

18. This emphasis on realism is particularly striking given the widespread panic that ensued in response to the original Orson Welles radio broadcast of *The War of the Worlds* in 1938. The radio play was presented as a live emergency report of a real invasion of the earth by flying saucers, and the persuasiveness of the performance was produced through the very type of journalistic authority that covers over the lack of visible evidence in public health films.

19. The local psychiatrist explains this series of events as "A strange neurosis, evidently contagious, an epidemic mass hysteria. In two weeks it's spread all over town," caused by, "worry about what's going on in the world, probably." However, the authority of this diagnosis is shortly undermined by the revelation that the psychiatrist himself is part of the alien conspiracy.

20. By comparing a popular book that functions as an exemplary diagnosis of the 1950s, from the 1950s—David Riesman's *The Lonely Crowd*—with *Invasion of the Body Snatchers*, Stuart Samuels argues that the same personality types that Riesman identifies with the mass conformity of 1950s culture are reflected in the film. Samuels, "The Age of Conspiracy and Conformity," 208. See Riesman, *The Lonely Crowd*. See also the anthology *Invasion of the Body Snatchers*, which collects the film's continuity script, postproduction file, and critical essays, and in which the editor argues that *Invasion* has "a central theme that is foregrounded: the fear of social conformity and the loss of self that results from it." LaValley, *Invasion of the Body Snatchers*, 4.

21. In his classic essay on the film, Stuart Samuels observes that, "Conspiracy theories feed off the idea of the normal being deceptive. In *Invasion*, the pods, the alien invaders, take on the appearance of normal people. It becomes physically impossible to tell the difference between the aliens and the normals." Samuels, "The Age of Conspiracy and Conformity," 209. Similarly, Michael Rogin has theorized the anxiety about invisible invasions of bodily borders from within the discourse of anti-Communism: "The pods in *Body Snatchers* and the people implanted with electronic control devices in *Invaders from Mars* alienate their families by pretending still to be themselves. Reds were visibly alien in earlier Red scares; they were the others. They moved inside our minds and bodies in the 1950s, and one could not tell them from anyone else. The vulnerability of the self to influence, upon which domestic ideology had hoped to capitalize, resulted in Communist influence instead. Surveillance and inquisition exposed domestic forces that had taken possession of the nation and

the self. No longer part of a conflict between contrasting classes, 1950s Communists were the invisible members of (and thereby exposed anxieties about) American mass society." Rogin, *Ronald Reagan, the Movie and Other Episodes in Political Demonology*, 267.

22. Sayre, *Running Time*, 201.

23. Seed, *American Science Fiction and the Cold War*, 133–34. The sources of the citations within Seed's quote are Weart, *Nuclear Fear*, 189–90; LaValley, *Invasion of the Body Snatchers*, 48; Peary, *Cult Movies*, 157; Warren, *Keep Watching the Skies!*

24. Rogin, *Ronald Reagan, the Movie and Other Episodes in Political Demonology*, 238.

25. R. Williams, *Television*.

26. For more on this topic, see Morse, "An Ontology of Everyday Distraction."

27. Kinsey and the Institute for Sex Research, *Sexual Behavior in the Human Male* and *Sexual Behavior in the Human Female*.

28. Rogin, *Ronald Reagan, the Movie and Other Episodes in Political Demonology*, 267. Similarly, Nancy Steffen-Fluhr argues that the pods are unconsciously tapping patriarchal myths about reproduction and female genitalia, the female body as the locus of death, new life, and an overall dangerous fecundity. Steffen-Fluhr, "Women and the Inner Game of Don Siegel's *Invasion of the Body Snatchers*."

29. While these networks traversed the globe long before World War Two, their transnational range acquired an intensified discursive prominence in the postwar period. See Mattelart, *Networking the World, 1794–2000*; Hills, *The Struggle for Control of Global Communication*; Whalen, *The Origins of Satellite Communications, 1945–1965*. On the intersections of human migration patterns and the global spread of disease, see Diamond, *Guns, Germs, and Steel*.

30. The television series *The Invaders* (1967–68) rehearsed this problematic week after week; the hero, architect David Vincent, has seen the alien invaders, but each time he discovers concrete, visible evidence that will convince the authorities that he's not insane and Earth really *has* been invaded, the proof disappears before it can be witnessed by an authorized gaze.

31. *It Came from Outer Space* was originally released as a three-dimensional film, although the effect is no longer apparent when viewed on vhs or dvd. Thus, the use of point-of-view camerawork would have been even more obvious to viewers in the 1950s, who (theoretically) would have experienced such shots as if the alien were looking right at them.

32. Later, this trope becomes the source of satire; in the 1967 parody of conspiracy films, *The President's Analyst* (1967), the telephone company ends up controlling the world and plotting to assassinate the president of the United States.

33. See chapter 1 for a discussion of the Payne Fund Studies and "emotional possession."

34. As Patrick Lucanio has noted, "A definite sign of America's advancing space technology in the fifties was the Palomar Observatory atop Palomar Mountain in Southern California. With its 200-inch Hale telescope, Palomar made headlines as a mighty stride in technology and astronomy." Lucanio, *Them or Us*, 71–72.

35. Moreover, the genre is rife with such gender stereotypes as the virile male scientist

and the subservient, bespectacled female assistant. See Doane, "Film and the Masquerade," in *Femmes Fatales* for a discussion of the relationship between sexuality, vision, and "the woman with glasses." See Sobchack, *Screening Space* for a thorough review of the representational conventions in science fiction films.

36. On the linkage of sexuality and "moral panics," see Rubin, "Thinking Sex"; Weeks, *Sex, Politics, and Society*; and D'Emilio, *Sexual Politics, Sexual Communities*. On sexual themes underlying apparent Communist paranoia in the Cold War films of Alfred Hitchcock, see Corber, *In the Name of National Security*.

37. Amusingly, in *It Conquered the World*, the extra bodies are actually put to work repairing the broken-down spaceship. In *I Married a Monster from Outer Space*, the bodies hang lifeless inside of the spaceship, attached to "an electronic broadcasting device." And in *Invasion of the Body Snatchers*, the extra bodies are the pods that occupy the liminal spaces of the film, in varying stages of development, waiting for the victim to sleep so they can take its place.

38. While both male and female bodily boundaries are "penetrated" in many of these films, the male possession is always the event that drives the narrative, the crisis that demands resolution.

39. Foucault, *The History of Sexuality, Volume I*, 69.

40. Sedgwick, *Epistemology of the Closet*, 80.

41. For a discussion of how the "homosexual panic" defense plays out in u.s. courtrooms, see Bagnall, "Burdens on Gay Litigants and Bias in the Court System." See also Sedgwick, *Between Men*; and Butler, "Contagious Word," in *Excitable Speech*.

42. This sequence also epitomizes the widespread attribution of "feminizing" effects to the other prominent "set" that was interfering with domestic harmony in this period, namely, the television set. For a discussion of the gender effects attributed to television viewing see Spigel, *Make Room for TV*.

43. Sedgwick, *Epistemology of the Closet*, 75.

44. For other interpretations of the sexual implications of "x" marking the site of implantation or bodily border penetration, see Sobchack, "The Virginity of Astronauts." See also Knee, *The American Science Fiction Film and Fifties Culture*, 193–99.

45. And yet, despite the importance of polio to the mid-century pursuit of public health in the United States, my research uncovered very few public health films on this topic. This relative absence may be explained in part by the support of Hollywood studios and stars for charity organizations that raised funds to fight the disease; more extensive research might uncover a collection of polio films in a Hollywood studio archive, rather than in the medical film collections where the research for this book was conducted.

46. For analysis of the gender dynamics in *I Married a Monster from Outer Space*, see Knee, *The American Science Fiction Film and Fifties Culture*; and Hendershot, *Paranoia, the Bomb, and 1950s Science Fiction Films*. After World War Two ended, many women who had left the domestic sphere in order to run the factories that supplied wartime munitions were

fired from their jobs, but many didn't want to return to being housewives, thus producing the widely noted gender struggles of this period. For more on this historical context, see Meyerowitz, *Not June Cleaver*, and E. T. May, *Homeward Bound*.

47. See Lisa Cartwright's fascinating discussion of the social dissemination of X-ray technology in the 1950s, in *Screening the Body*.

48. This scenario further enacts Foucault's claim that "we demand that sex speak the truth . . . and we demand that it tell us our truth, or rather, the deeply buried truth of that truth about ourselves which we think we possess in our immediate consciousness." Foucault, *The History of Sexuality*, 69.

49. Knee, *The American Science Fiction Film and Fifties Culture*, 405.

50. Ibid., 405–6.

51. See Curtin and Spigel, *The Revolution Wasn't Televised*; Gitlin, *The Whole World Is Watching*; Branch, *Parting the Waters*; J. Williams, *Eyes on the Prize*.

52. The importance of understanding this constellation of discourses in the postwar period as addressing issues other than (or at least, in addition to) Communism becomes apparent when a supposed Communist invasion allegory of the period, such as *Invasion of the Body Snatchers* (1956), is compared with a later anti-Communist film that would, under the allegory explanation, be part of the same genre, such as *Red Dawn* (1984). The notable lack of imagery of bodily invasion and contagion in the later film highlights the extent to which, at the very least, there is more than Communist paranoia at work in the earlier film and its mode of representing invasion.

4 CONSPIRACY AND CARTOGRAPHY

1. World Health Organization, *Introducing WHO*, 8. See also the chronology in K. Lee, *Historical Dictionary of the World Health Organization*, xxiii.

2. 1851 was also the year that the first undersea telegraph cable was laid. See Mattelart, *Networking the World*, 11. On the intersecting histories of public health and immigration, see Kraut, *Silent Travelers*; R. C. Williams, *The United States Public Health Service*; Duffy, *The Sanitarians*; and Wolf, *Europe and the People Without History*.

3. Thrower, *Maps and Civilization*, 150–52.

4. Similarly, the ability to identify specific causes of disease that developed with the "bacteriological revolution" of the 1880s did not prevent the continued attribution of contagion to racial and ethnic "others."

5. Ibid., 152. See also Allan Sekula's excellent essay, "The Body and the Archive."

6. A key figure in the early history of documentary cinema, Robert J. Flaherty—the renowned director of *Nanook of the North* (1922)—was engaged simultaneously in capturing images of native "others" in exotic locales and in exploration and cartography. See Flaherty, "The Belcher Islands of Hudson Bay." See also Fatimah Tobing Rony's discussion of Flaherty's work in *The Third Eye*.

7. It was not only immigrants who were perceived as vectors of alien contagions; any

bodies that traveled beyond u.s. borders were suspect—this included merchant seamen and u.s. soldiers in the Spanish American War and World Wars I and II. The surgeon general's *Annual Report* of 1878 revealed that at least 40 percent of American seamen were carriers of venereal disease. Mullan, *Plagues and Politics*, 29. This observation, based on statistics from the Marine Hospital Service, highlights the linkage of global commerce and sexuality from the early days of institutionalized public health—a linkage that becomes more prominent in anti–venereal disease public health film campaigns directed at soldiers during World War One. By World War Two, as demonstrated by *Hemolytic Streptococcus Control* (1945), this linkage becomes even more hyperbolic; public health films of the later period posit a causal link between the sexual implications of the homosocial armed services and the spread of contagious diseases.

8. World Health Organization, *Introducing who*, 8–16; R. C. Williams, *The United States Public Health Service*, 441–42; see also Brockington, *World Health*.

9. Etheridge, *Sentinel for Health*, xv–xvi.

10. R. C. Williams, *The United States Public Health Service*, 398.

11. Etheridge, *Sentinel for Health*, 24.

12. Ibid., 56.

13. G. King, *Mapping Reality*, 26.

14. Duffy, *The Sanitarians*, 279.

15. Mullan, *Plagues and Politics*, 139.

16. R. C. Williams, *The United States Public Health Service*, 401.

17. A crucial—and rare—source of information about the wide distribution and exhibition of public health films is the work of Adolf Nichtenhauser, an early promoter of motion pictures as medical and public health training tools. See Nichtenhauser, "A History of Motion Pictures in Medicine."

18. Etheridge, *Sentinel for Health*, 7.

19. R. C. Williams, *The United States Public Health Service*, 402.

20. Ibid., 407. The popular visibility of institutions of public health in this period is perhaps best represented by the massive nationwide polio immunization drives of the early 1960s, which were assisted by film campaigns using Hollywood stars to promote vaccination and charitable giving. See Gould, *A Summer Plague*, 85.

21. Etheridge, *Sentinel for Health*, 111.

22. Thrower, *Maps and Civilization*, 200.

23. Etheridge, *Sentinel for Health*, 135.

24. Watson, *The Expanding Vista*, 22. For a discussion of the ideological implications of this shift in television programming, see Curtin, *Redeeming the Wasteland*; and Lentz, "*Quality* versus *Relevance*."

25. For a history of cartography that includes some reference to epidemiology, see Thrower, *Maps and Civilization*.

26. G. King, *Mapping Reality*, 25–26; Wood, *The Power of Maps*, 4–5. See Althusser, "Ide-

ology and Ideological State Apparatuses (Notes toward an Investigation)." Wood continues: "This, essentially, is what maps give us, *reality*, a reality that exceeds our vision, our reach, the span of our days, a reality we achieve no other way. We are always mapping the invisible or the unattainable or the erasable, the future or the past, the whatever-is-not-here-present-to-our-senses-now and, through the gift that the map gives us, transmuting it into everything it is not . . . *into the real*" (emphasis in original). In his influential work, *Understanding Media*, Marshall McLuhan points out that "it is usually forgotten that without prints and blueprints, without maps and geometry, the world of modern sciences and techniques would hardly exist." McLuhan, *Understanding Media*, 157. For an analysis of the ideological work of mapping practices, see Monmonier, *How to Lie with Maps*. On the intersections of cartography and theories of the nation and nationality, see Hobsbawm, *Nations and Nationalism Since 1780*; B. Anderson, *Imagined Communities*; and Bhabha, *Nation and Narration*.

27. In *Maps and Politics* (1997), Jeremy Black introduces his critique of the presumed objectivity of maps through reference to the work of Michel Foucault, who, Black argues, "sought to use the notions, symbols and language of cartography, specifically of space, boundaries and networks, in order to understand and make dynamic his views on the politics of knowledge. For Foucault, knowledge as struggle was to be understood in large part by reference to space: there were boundaries and spheres of contest; ideologies colonized terrains." In turn, Black notes that Foucault's own work, along with that of other poststructuralist theorists such as Roland Barthes, Jacques Derrida, and Henri Lefebvre, has influenced the field of cartography. Ibid., 18, 65. See Foucault, *Discipline and Punish*. See also Denis Wood's extended discussion of mapping practices in terms of Roland Barthes's semiotic analysis of "myths," especially chapter 5, "The Interest Is Embodied in the Map in Signs and Myths," in *The Power of Maps*. See also Barthes, *Mythologies*, *Camera Lucida*, and "The Plates of the Encyclopedia." See also Lefebvre, *The Production of Space*.

28. Baudrillard, *Simulations*, 2.

29. G. King, *Mapping Reality*, 78. In this passage, King is introducing his discussion of several widely read and influential analyses of the postwar period, including Boorstin's *The Image*, Packard's *The Hidden Persuaders*, and DeBord's *Society of the Spectacle*. However, in a discussion of the work of Jean Baudrillard and Umberto Eco, King makes the important corrective historical point that, "This kind of dialectic between real and fake, authentic and copy, is far from new. A similar tension was felt in the second half of the nineteenth century, for example, when the new possibilities for imitation and illusion created by technological developments in the fabrication of materials provoked demands for a return to a real or an authentic believed to be threatened with displacement." G. King, *Mapping Reality*, 87. See Eco, *Travels in Hyperreality*. See also Orvell, *The Real Thing*.

30. The most prominent literary examples include the work of Thomas Pynchon, Don DeLillo, Kathy Acker, Ishmael Reed, Philip K. Dick, Joseph Heller, Norman Mailer, and Margaret Atwood, to name a few. Conspiracy theories relating to the Cold War and especially to the assassination of John F. Kennedy are too numerous to list here, but a foun-

dational overview can be found in Hofstadter, *The Paranoid Style in American Politics and Other Essays.* Cultural theorists who address paranoia and conspiracy include Jameson, Foucault, Baudrillard, Deleuze and Guattari, Polan, O'Donnell, Melley, Fenster, S. Miller, and more. Many of these refer back to the psychoanalytic treatment of these topics by Freud and Lacan.

31. Melley, *Empire of Conspiracy*, 13, 7–8.

32. Fenster, *Conspiracy Theories*, 80. Fenster goes on to note: "Based on a circular drive to find the 'truth'—a kind of epistemophilia—. . . [conspiracy theory] becomes akin to the Lacanian notion of desire, which requires, at its core, that its ultimate fulfillment be continually deferred." Ibid., 89. Similarly, Patrick O'Donnell describes cultural paranoia as "a mode of perception that notes the connectedness between things in a hyperbolic metonymizing of reality." O'Donnell, "Engendering Paranoia in Contemporary Narrative," 181.

33. G. King, *Mapping Reality*, 52. This movement works as "a process of 'deterritorialization,' as Gilles Deleuze and Felix Guattari put it, in which the surface of the map is rendered blurred and slippery, followed by one of 'reterritorialization,' when new grid references are inscribed." Ibid., 57. See Deleuze and Guattari, *Anti-Oedipus*.

34. "Injection panic" scenes take place in *Panic in the Streets* (1950), *The Andromeda Strain* (1971), *The Crazies* (1973), and *Outbreak* (1995), and in such public health films as *Prevention of the Introduction of Diseases from Abroad* (1945), *The Eternal Fight* (1948), and *A Monthly Review from Europe* (1952).

35. Melley, *Empire of Conspiracy*, 32. Italics in original.

36. Ibid., 32–33.

37. Melley specifically references Baudrillard's "The Ecstasy of Communication."

38. See Mary Ann Doane's discussion of the "problem" of female spectatorship as an "overpresence of the image," wherein the impossibility of achieving spatial distance "prevents the woman from assuming a position similar to the man's in relation to signifying systems." Doane, "Film and the Masquerade," in *Femmes Fatales*, 22–23.

39. Melley, *Empire of Conspiracy*, 33.

40. For a development of this argument, see Huyssen, "Mass Culture as Woman."

41. See Philip Wylie, *Generation of Vipers* and Sloan Wilson, *The Man in the Gray Flannel Suit*. Kaja Silverman analyzes this shift in "Historical Trauma and Male Subjectivity." See also Cohan and Hark, *Screening the Male*; Penley and Willis, *Male Trouble*.

42. See Eberwein, *Sex Ed* for additional discussion of *Fight Syphilis*.

43. Similarly, the centrality of surveillance technologies to the practice of public health is also emphasized in a segment of *Prevention of the Introduction of Diseases from Abroad*, titled, "Keeping Currently Informed on the Prevalence of Disease." Over a global map with dots marking the sites of epidemiological surveillance, the voiceover explains that the USPHS "maintains an intelligence office regarding the occurrence of epidemic diseases in the United States and foreign countries, and reports are received weekly from all American consulates." This claim is accompanied by a montage of communications networks,

including the telegraph and postal service connecting domestic and foreign consulates to the surgeon general's office at the USPHS.

44. For another example of epidemiology as detective story, see *Public Health: A Case of the Blues* (n.d.).

45. It is significant that the disease is known as "Asian" influenza, while the pandemic of 1918 is not usually remembered as "Spanish" influenza, despite the purported origins of the outbreak in that country. The selective use of incriminating appellations underscores the ideological, rather than scientific, function of such terms and seriously undermines any claims of epidemiological objectivity invoked in their defense. For a discussion of representations of "Asians" in popular culture, see R. Lee, *Orientals*; Marchetti, *Romance and the Yellow Peril*; and Eng, *Racial Castration*.

5 INDEXICAL DIGITAL

1. This formulation has functioned as common sense in film theory since Laura Mulvey published her groundbreaking essay "Visual Pleasure and Narrative Cinema" in 1975. While many of Mulvey's claims about female spectatorship were criticized and revised in subsequent years, her most basic assertions concerning the active and passive gender dichotomies in mainstream cinema continue to be treated as axiomatic.

2. Neale, "Masculinity as Spectacle," 19.

3. See Corber, *Homosexuality in Cold War America*.

4. By "profilmic" I mean "The physical material of the scene prior to the act of filming" or, in other words, what is in front of the camera, about to be shot on film. Stam, Burgoyne, and Flitterman-Lewis, *New Vocabularies in Film Semiotics*, 112.

5. The film explains Hall's positioning through the "Robertson Odd Man Hypothesis" (invented by Michael Crichton, author of the original novel, *The Andromeda Strain*), which concludes that "an unmarried male should carry out command decisions involving thermonuclear destruct contexts."

6. On televisual "liveness," see Feuer, "The Concept of Live Television"; Stam, "Television News and Its Spectator"; Doane, "Information, Crisis, Catastrophe"; and Morse, "The Television News Personality and Credibility."

7. See Lacan, *Écrits*; and Derrida, "Différance." Technophilic or phobic conspiracy films are driven by the desire to reunite the audiovisual representation with the body that it represents. For instance, in *Blow Out* (1981) and *The Conversation* (1974) the search for the bodily source of the recorded sounds is a search for access to the "real," to discover or attain an unmediated relationship to reality, which is increasingly impossible in mass-mediated, late-twentieth-century culture. This search for bodily integrity can be seen as a search for coherent subjectivity, an attempt to return to a moment prior to fractured subjectivity.

8. This reaction is itself characteristic of (if implicit in) the work of numerous theorists of postmodernity, whose analyses of conspiracy belie a widely noted masculinist fear of bodily absorption into the feminized realm of image-based mass culture and globalization. The

totalizing view of postmodernity as a simulacral system producing depthless subjectivity construes the implicitly masculine subject as vulnerable to contamination by the excessive proximity between the image and the "self." But the anxiety that theorists like Jean Baudrillard attach to the advent of postmodernity is far from new; rather, it is only the latest version of a highly gendered form of anxiety about the impact of mass cultural technologies of reproduction on individual subjectivity. For a development of this argument, see Huyssen, "Mass Culture as Woman."

9. On the collapse of anal eroticism and death, see Bersani, "Is the Rectum a Grave?"; and D. A. Miller, "Anal Rope."

10. See Sedgwick, *Between Men* and *Epistemology of the Closet*.

11. For additional examples of this form of narrative nonclosure, see *Three Days of the Condor* (1975) and *The Parallax View* (1974).

12. The foundational text on the integration of bodies and machines is Haraway, *Simians, Cyborgs and Women*. See also Springer, *Electronic Eros*; Balsamo, *Technologies of the Gendered Body*.

13. Neale, "Masculinity as Spectacle," 14.

14. Duffy, *The Sanitarians*, 300.

15. Numerous texts have been written on specific aspects of each of these events. A useful collection of essays is Bernstein, *Controlling Hollywood*. For a good overview, see Thompson and Bordwell, *Film History* and D. Cook, *A History of Narrative Film*.

16. *Guess Who's Coming to Dinner?* (1967) was considered by many to be a groundbreaking film in its liberal treatment of interracial marriage, but it was also widely seen as assimilationist and therefore politically conservative.

17. *Sweet Sweetback's Baadasssss Song* (1971) and *Shaft* (1971).

18. Guerrero, *Framing Blackness*, 70.

19. The major critiques were that the films were regressive in their treatment of gender and that they ultimately celebrated a ghetto pimp style without any political content, thus perpetuating rather than undermining negative stereotypes about African Americans. For an excellent analysis of both sides of the debate, see Isaac Julien's documentary, *BaadAssss Cinema* (2002). See also Lev, *American Films of the '70s*.

20. Guerrero, *Framing Blackness*, 113.

21. Guerrero calls this cycle the "original black cinema paradox," which he characterizes as follows: "Hollywood . . . employs a mixed bag of tricks and strategies to contain any challenge to its cinematic regime, according to its needs at a given historical moment. Thus the studio system is quite adept at containing insurgent impulses of difference, usually by excluding or ignoring them, but also in times of economic insecurity or shifting cultural relations by the more pervasive strategy of co-opting resistant images and narratives into the vast metamorphosing body of its cinematic hegemony. Thus a black director may make the most popular film ever or successfully work a very lucrative genre only to find that the studio system has co-opted the form of blackness while emptying it of its emancipatory content and cultural impact." Ibid., 182.

22. The classic and definitive elaboration of this concept in the field of anthropology is M. Douglas, *Purity and Danger*.

23. Kinsella, *Covering the Plague*. See also Patton, *Sex and Germs*; Watney, *Policing Desire*; Crimp, *AIDS*; Treichler, *How to Have Theory in an Epidemic*; Patton, *Inventing AIDS*; and Crimp, *Melancholia and Moralism*.

24. James Kinsella cites the successes of playwright Larry Kramer and the protest group ACT-UP (AIDS Coalition to Unleash Power) in securing mass media coverage of AIDS and in changing the plotline of a homophobic TV drama called *Midnight Caller*. Kinsella, *Covering the Plague*, 257.

25. Bordwell and Thompson, *Film Art*, 19. For a brief overview of the demise of educational filmmaking dated here at 1985, see the "Fact Sheet" on the Web site of the Academic Film Archive of North America, http://www.afana.org/facts.htm. Many thanks to Geoff Alexander for providing useful information about researching educational films.

26. Although the early 1960s was a period of extensive primetime documentary programming on network television, it wasn't until the mid-1970s that the newsmagazine became an influential format. The genre was initially dominated by the success of *60 Minutes* on CBS, but during the 1980s, reality programming dramatically expanded on the networks and cable. Programming included *20/20*, *Entertainment Tonight*, *Unsolved Mysteries*, *America's Most Wanted*, *A Current Affair*, and *The People's Court*. In the same period, the subgenre of talk television exploded, with programs like *The Oprah Winfrey Show*, *The Donahue Show*, and *Geraldo*. On 1960s television documentaries, see Curtin, *Redeeming the Wasteland*. On *60 Minutes*, see R. Campbell, "Securing the Middle Ground." On reality programming in the 1980s, see Barnouw, *Tube of Plenty*, 519–22, and Friedman, *Reality Squared*, 1.

27. Juhasz, *AIDS TV*. See note 23.

28. For an extended discussion of the legal discourse of acts versus identities, focusing on the Supreme Court decision in *Bowers v. Hardwick* and its impact on gay communities, see Sedgwick, *Epistemology of the Closet*, 86–90.

29. *Can AIDS Be Stopped?* (1986) employs a similar strategy, including an animated globe that circles, first centering on Africa, then turning to Europe, with infected countries highlighted in red and special emphasis on cities that have a high population of homosexuals and intravenous drug users. And in *AIDS: The Surgeon General's Update* (1987), a voiceover notes that "With the mobility of our society, AIDS will spread everywhere" over an animated globe with lit-up hot spots. Again, in *The AIDS Quarterly* (1990): "You cannot really build a fence around a community—any community of any size—they couldn't do it in the plagues in Europe, and they can't do it in this major epidemic in our country." In contrast, *Our Immune System* (1988) assures viewers that "vaccination against harmful microorganisms from distant places has made travel much safer." Other AIDS videos that use the animated globe technique include *About AIDS* (1986), *AIDS . . . What YOU Need to Know* (1987), *AIDS: The Surgeon General's Update* (1987), *The AIDS Quarterly* (1990), *The Coming Plague* (1997).

30. While it is important to recognize the effectiveness of activist strategies here, it is

equally important to acknowledge their shortcomings. For a thorough discussion of the various failures of both AIDS activists and the mass media, see Patton, *Fatal Advice*.

31. Hart, *The AIDS Movie*, xi.

32. For commentary on viral rhetoric in a discussion of the politics of computer hacking, see Ross, "Hacking Away at the Counterculture."

33. Robin Cook's novel titled *Outbreak* is only thematically related to the later eponymous film. See also the slightly less recent Regis, *Virus Ground Zero*; and Lundell, *Virus!*

34. Russell Watson, "Why Viruses Push Our Hot Buttons," *Newsweek*, May 22, 1995, 54.

35. Richard Preston, "Crisis in the Hot Zone," *New Yorker*, October 26, 1992, 62.

36. See Treichler, "AIDS Narrative on Television," 163. See also Browning, *Infectious Rhythm*.

37. Laurie Garrett, "Plague Warriors," *Vanity Fair*, August 1995, 86.

38. Preston, "Crisis in the Hot Zone," 62. Bernard Weinraub, "Two Films, One Subject. Uh-Oh. In Hollywood, the Race Is On," *New York Times*, June 23, 1994, C11.

39. Bernard Weinraub, "Wrestling a Virus to the Screen," *New York Times*, March 19, 1995, C14. Robert W. Welkos, "Success of Warner's 'Outbreak' Spreads," *Los Angeles Times*, March 21, 1995, C32. Jeannette Walls, "Paging Dr. Angelou," *Esquire*, May 1995, 32.

40. Preston, *The Hot Zone*, 243–44.

41. The representation of the horror of the Ebola outbreaks always returns to the African medical workers' "unsafe" treatment procedures: they don't have latex gloves, they reuse needles, they touch the patient's blood with their bare hands. As with AIDS, the site of contamination expands from "African" bodies with Ebola to encompass the entire continent. "Africa" becomes a dirty, infectious, "premodern" world, in contrast to the medical and technological superiority of the United States, thus effectively denying the U.S. government's institutionalized neglect of people with HIV and AIDS.

42. Preston, "Crisis in the Hot Zone," 58–60, 70, 79.

43. Preston, *The Hot Zone*, 204.

44. Ibid., 223.

45. Preston, "Crisis in the Hot Zone," 68.

46. The same representational strategies were used in coverage of the spring 2003 global severe acute respiratory syndrome (SARS) outbreak. For example, an article on the cover of the Sunday, April 27, 2003, *New York Times* was titled "From China's Provinces, A Crafty Germ Breaks Out" and placed over a large color photograph with the heading, "Workers prepared wild game hens on the floor of a restaurant in Guangzhou, China. Food workers were among the earliest SARS patients."

47. For an excellent discussion of the racialized regimes of visuality that treat "whiteness" as an invisible signifier while "blackness" is collapsed with "race," see Dyer, "White." See also Dyer's book-length study of the topic, *White*.

48. Casey is pictured casually reclining, eating a candy bar, reading a magazine, humming and tapping his foot along to music playing on his Walkman, as the USAMRIID crew flies into "the hot zone" in the Motaba River Valley, Zaire.

49. *The Wizard of Oz* (1939).

50. In *AIDS: Everything You and Your Family Need to Know . . . But Were Afraid to Ask* (1988), Surgeon General C. Everett Koop claims that "the AIDS problem started in African monkeys," despite the lack of epidemiological evidence confirming that statement.

51. Patton, *Inventing AIDS*, 78.

52. At this point in the narrative, "Motaba" has penetrated the United States and claimed three victims. The epidemic is about to begin. In the chain of contaminating transnational commerce outlined thus far, an African monkey, illegally imported to the United States, has infected two people (through saliva and blood). A transcontinental airplane flight later, the importer kisses and infects his girlfriend, and they both die within twenty-four hours without infecting anyone else. Meanwhile, the pet shop owner who was scratched by the monkey collapses in convulsions and is rushed to the hospital, where a medical intern takes a blood sample. As he spins the blood samples in a centrifuge, the intern lifts the lid of the machine and sticks his hand inside, while the glass vials are still spinning. The glass breaks, blood sprays everywhere, and he is infected. Later that night, the intern and his girlfriend go to the movies.

53. For a fascinating discussion of global maps depicting Internet use and access that draw on "visual discourses of identity and negated identity that echo those of European maps of colonized and colonizable space of nearly a century ago," see Harpold, "Dark Continents," 5. Harpold links the "exploration" of the Internet, the global expansion of telecommunications corporations, and discourses of colonialism: "In a deeply ironic way, the networked instauration of the dark continent reverses the extractive logic of classic colonialism: instead of raw materials (ore, precious stones, humans) freighted out of the heart of darkness for consumption by the wired-colonial metropole, the information order, to the extent that it penetrates the unwired world, will be largely devoted to freighting information in its motley forms into the benighted realms. In this context, 'information' has the sense of both a commodity—a thing for sale over the networks—and a coercive force: the networks are able to inform the unwired realms; the new dark continent reproduces itself over the wires without regard for the prior conventional definitions of nation, region, or continent." Ibid., 19–20.

54. The majority of the AIDS education videos insert still documentary photographs into the narrative at some point, to underscore their truth value and objectivity. See for example *AIDS Hits Home* (1986), *AIDS: Changing the Rules* (1987), *AIDS* (1987), *An Epidemic of Fear* (1987), *AIDS: Everything You and Your Family Need to Know . . . But Were Afraid to Ask* (1988), *Our Immune System* (1988), *Growing Up in the Age of AIDS* (1992), *The Coming Plague* (1997).

CONCLUSION

1. Yoshimoto, "Real Virtuality," 111.

2. As Andrew Ross has noted, "The epidemiology of *biological* virus (especially AIDS) research is being studied closely to help implement *computer* security plans" (emphasis mine). Ross, "Hacking Away at the Counterculture," 248.

3. "Attack of the Love Bug," *Time*, May 15, 2000, 49.

4. Kolko, Nakamura, and Rodman, eds. *Race in Cyberspace*, 1.

5. Turkle, *Life on the Screen*, 211.

6. "Attack of the Love Bug," 52.

7. This is not to suggest that such crimes have not been committed, but rather to highlight the prevalence of sexual imagery in popular Internet rhetoric.

8. "Privacy Questions Raised in Cases of Syphilis Linked to Chat Room," *New York Times*, August 25, 1999, A1.

9. Manovich, "The Paradoxes of Digital Photography."

10. For an excellent critique of the rhetoric of "new" media, see P. Rosen, "Old and New."

11. For discussions of the visual representation of AIDS, especially in relation to Africa, see the work of Cindy Patton, cited above, as well as Treichler, "AIDS, Africa, and Cultural Theory"; and Watney, "Missionary Positions."

Bibliography

Addams, Jane. *The Spirit of Youth and the City Streets*. New York: Macmillan, 1909.

Adler, Mortimer J. *Art and Prudence: A Study in Practical Philosophy*. New York: Longman, 1937.

Althusser, Louis. "Ideology and Ideological States Apparatuses (Notes Toward an Investigation)." In *Lenin and Philosophy, and Other Essays*. Trans. Ben Brewster. New York: Monthly Review, 1971.

Altman, Rick, ed. *Sound Theory/Sound Practice*. New York: Routledge, 1992.

Anderson, Benedict. *Imagined Communities: Reflections on the Origin and Spread of Nationalism*. New York: Verso, 1983.

Anderson, Milton. *The Modern Goliath*. Los Angeles: David, 1935.

Anzaldúa, Gloria. *Borderlands/La Frontera: The New Mestiza*. San Francisco: Aunt Lute, 1987.

Arthur, Paul. "Jargons of Authenticity (Three American Moments)." In *Theorizing Documentary*. Ed. by Michael Renov. New York: Routledge, 1993.

Bagnall, Robert G. "Burdens on Gay Litigants and Bias in the Court System: Homosexual Panic, Child Custody, and Anonymous Parties." *Harvard Civil Rights-Civil Liberties Law Review* 19 (summer 1984): 497–559.

Balio, Tino, ed. *Grand Design: Hollywood as a Modern Business Enterprise 1930–1939*. New York: Scribner's, 1993.

Balio, Tino, ed. *Hollywood in the Age of Television.* Cambridge: Unwin Hyman, 1990.

Balsamo, Anne. *Technologies of the Gendered Body: Reading Cyborg Women.* Durham: Duke University Press, 1996.

Barnouw, Eric. *Documentary: A History of the Non-Fiction Film.* New York: Oxford University Press, 1974.

———. *Tube of Plenty: The Evolution of American Television.* 2nd ed. New York: Oxford University Press, 1990.

Barthes, Roland. *Camera Lucida.* New York: Hill and Wang, 1981.

———. *Mythologies.* New York: Hill and Wang, 1972.

———. "The Plates of the Encyclopedia." In *New Critical Essays.* New York: Hill and Wang, 1980.

Baudrillard, Jean. "The Ecstasy of Communication." Trans. John Johnston. In *The Anti-Aesthetic: Essays on Postmodern Culture.* Ed. by Hal Foster. Port Townsend, Wash.: Bay, 1983.

———. *Simulations.* New York: Semiotext[e], 1983.

Bazin, André. *What Is Cinema?* Trans. Hugh Gray. Berkeley: University of California Press, 1967.

Benjamin, Walter. "The Work of Art in the Age of Mechanical Reproduction." In *Illuminations: Essays and Reflections.* Ed. by Hannah Arendt. Trans. Harry Zohn. New York: Harcourt, 1968.

Benson, Michael. *Vintage Science Fiction Films, 1896–1949.* Jefferson, N.C.: McFarland, 1985.

Benveniste, Emile. *Problems in General Linguistics.* Coral Gables: University of Miami Press, 1971.

Bernardi, Daniel, ed. *The Birth of Whiteness: Race and the Emergence of U.S. Cinema.* New Brunswick: Rutgers University Press, 1996.

Bernstein, Matthew, ed. *Controlling Hollywood: Censorship and Regulation in the Studio Era.* New Brunswick: Rutgers University Press, 1999.

Bersani, Leo. "Is the Rectum a Grave?" *October* 43 (winter 1987): 197–222.

Bhabha, Homi, ed. *Nation and Narration.* New York: Routledge, 1990.

Biskind, Peter. *Seeing Is Believing: How Hollywood Taught Us to Stop Worrying and Love the Fifties.* New York: Pantheon, 1983.

Black, Gregory D. *Hollywood Censored: Morality Codes, Catholics, and the Movies.* New York: Cambridge University Press, 1994.

———. "Hollywood Censored: The Production Code Administration and the Hollywood Film Industry, 1930–1940." *Film History* 3, no. 3 (1989).

Black, Jeremy. *Maps and Politics.* Chicago: University of Chicago Press, 1997.

Blumer, Herbert. *Movies and Conduct.* New York: Macmillan, 1933.

Blumer, Herbert, and Philip M. Hauser. *Movies, Delinquency, and Crime.* New York: Macmillan, 1933.

Boorstin, Daniel. *The Image, or, What Happened to the American Dream.* New York: Atheneum, 1961.

Bordwell, David, and Kristin Thompson. *Film Art: An Introduction.* 5th ed. New York: McGraw-Hill, 1997.

Branch, Taylor. *Parting the Waters: America in the King Years, 1954–1963.* New York: Simon and Schuster, 1988.

Brandt, Allan M. *No Magic Bullet: A Social History of Venereal Disease in the United States Since 1880.* New York: Oxford University Press, 1987.

Braun, Marta. *Picturing Time: The Work of Etienne-Jules Maret.* Chicago: University of Chicago Press, 1992.

Brockington, Fraser. *World Health.* New York: Churchill Livingstone, 1975.

Brown, JoAnne. "Crime, Commerce, and Contagionism: The Political Languages of Public Health and the Popularization of Germ Theory in the United States, 1870–1950." In *Scientific Authority and Twentieth-Century America.* Ed. by Ronald G. Walters. Baltimore: Johns Hopkins University Press, 1997.

Browning, Barbara. *Infectious Rhythm: Metaphors of Contagion and the Spread of African Culture.* New York: Routledge, 1998.

Brunstetter, M. R. *How to Use the Educational Sound Film.* Chicago: University of Chicago Press, 1937.

Butler, Judith. *Excitable Speech: A Politics of the Performative.* New York: Routledge, 1997.

Caldwell, John Thornton, ed. *Electronic Media and Technoculture.* New Brunswick: Rutgers University Press, 2000.

Campbell, Craig. *Reel America and World War I.* London: McFarland, 1985.

Campbell, Richard. "Securing the Middle Ground: Reporter Formulas in 60 Minutes." In *Television: The Critical View.* 5th ed. Ed. by Horace Newcomb. New York: Oxford University Press, 1994.

Cartwright, Lisa. *Screening the Body: Tracing Medicine's Visual Culture*. Minneapolis: University of Minnesota Press, 1995.

Castonguay, James. "The Spanish American War in u.s. Media Culture." In *American Quarterly*. "Hypertext Scholarship in American Studies." Crossroads Project. http://chnm.gmu.edu/aq/war. 1999.

Caughie, John, ed. *Theories of Authorship: A Reader*. New York: Routledge, 1986.

Charters, W. W. *Motion Pictures and Youth: A Summary*. New York: Macmillan, 1933.

Chauncey, George. "Christian Brotherhood or Sexual Perversion? Homosexual Identities and the Construction of Sexual Boundaries in the World War I Era." In *Gender and American History Since 1890*. Ed. by Barbara Melosh. New York: Routledge, 1992.

Chion, Michel. *Audio-Vision: Sound on Screen*. Trans. Claudia Gorbman. New York: Columbia University Press, 1994.

Cholodenko, Alan, ed. *The Illusion of Life: Essays on Animation*. Sydney: Southwood, 1991.

Chow, Rey. *Primitive Passions: Visuality, Sexuality, Ethnography and Contemporary Chinese Cinema*. New York: Columbia University Press, 1995.

Cohan, Steve, and Ina Rae Hark, eds. *Screening the Male: Exploring Masculinities in Hollywood Cinema*. New York: Routledge, 1993.

Comolli, Jean-Louis, and Jean Narboni. "Cinema/Ideology/Criticism." In *Screen Reader: Cinema/Ideology/Politics*. London: SEFT, 1977.

———. "Parenthesis or Indirect Route: An Attempt at Theoretical Definition of the Relationship between Cinema and Politics." In *Screen Reader: Cinema/Ideology/Politics*. London: SEFT, 1977.

Cook, David. *A History of Narrative Film*. 3rd ed. New York: Norton, 1996.

Cook, Robin. *Outbreak*. New York: Berkley, 1987.

Corber, Robert J. *Homosexuality in Cold War America: Resistance and the Crisis of Masculinity*. Durham: Duke University Press, 1997.

———. *In the Name of National Security: Hitchcock, Homophobia, and the Political Construction of Gender in Postwar America*. Durham: Duke University Press, 1993.

Corrigan, Timothy. *A Cinema Without Walls: Movies and Culture After Vietnam*. New Brunswick: Rutgers University Press, 1991.

Couvares, Francis G. "Hollywood, Main Street, and the Church: Trying to Censor the Movies Before the Production Code." *American Quarterly* 44, no. 4 (1992).

———, ed. *Movie Censorship and American Culture*. Washington: Smithsonian, 1996.

Crafton, Donald. *Before Mickey: The Animated Film, 1898–1928*. Cambridge: MIT Press, 1982.

Crary, Jonathan. *Techniques of the Observer: On Vision and Modernity in the Nineteenth Century*. Cambridge: MIT Press, 1990.

Crawford, Dorothy H. *The Invisible Enemy: A Natural History of Viruses*. New York: Oxford University Press, 2000.

Crimp, Douglas, ed. AIDS: *Cultural Analysis, Cultural Activism*. Cambridge: MIT Press, 1988.

———. *Melancholia and Moralism: Essays on* AIDS *and Queer Politics*. Cambridge: MIT Press, 2002.

Curtin, Michael. *Redeeming the Wasteland: Television Documentary and Cold War Politics*. New Brunswick: Rutgers University Press, 1995.

Curtin, Michael, and Lynn Spigel, eds. *The Revolution Wasn't Televised*. New York: Routledge, 1997.

Dale, Edgar. *Audiovisual Methods in Teaching*. New York: Dryden, 1946.

———. *Children's Attendance at Motion Pictures*. New York: Macmillan, 1933.

———. *The Content of Motion Pictures*. New York: Macmillan, 1933.

———. *How to Appreciate Motion Pictures*. New York: Macmillan, 1933.

Davies, Pete. *The Devil's Flu: The World's Deadliest Influenza Epidemic and the Scientific Hunt for the Virus That Caused It*. New York: Henry Holt, 2000.

Dean, Jodi. *Aliens in America: Conspiracy Cultures from Outerspace to Cyberspace*. Ithaca: Cornell University Press, 1998.

DeBauche, Leslie Midkiff. *Reel Patriotism: The Movies and World War I*. Madison: University of Wisconsin Press, 1997.

DeBord, Guy. *The Society of the Spectacle*. 1967. Trans. Donald Nicholson-Smith. New York: Zone, 1994.

DeCordova, Richard. *Picture Personalities: The Emergence of the Star System in America*. Urbana: University of Illinois Press, 1990.

Deleuze, Gilles, and Felix Guattari. *Anti-Oedipus: Capitalism and Schizophre-*

nia. 1972. Trans. Robert Hurley, Mark Seem, and Helen Lane. New York: Viking, 1977.

Delia, Jesse G. "Communication Research: A History." In *Handbook of Communication Sciences*. Ed. by Charles Berger and Steven H. Chaffee. Newbury Park, N.J.: Sage, 1987.

D'Emilio, John. *Sexual Politics, Sexual Communities: The Making of a Homosexual Minority in the United States, 1940–1970*. Chicago: University of Chicago Press, 1998.

Derrida, Jacques. "Différance." In *Speech and Phenomena*. Evanston, Ill.: Northwestern University Press, 1973.

Diamond, Jared. *Guns, Germs, and Steel: The Fates of Human Societies*. New York: Norton, 1997.

Dibbets, Karel, and Bert Hogenkamp, eds. *Film and the First World War*. Amsterdam: Amsterdam University Press, 1995.

Dinnerstein, Leonard, and David M. Reimers. *Ethnic Americans: A History of Immigration*. 4th ed. New York: Columbia University Press, 1999.

Doane, Mary Ann. *Femmes Fatales: Feminism, Film Theory, Psychoanalysis*. New York: Routledge, 1991.

———. "Information, Crisis, Catastrophe." In *Logics of Television: Essays in Cultural Criticism*. Ed. by Patricia Mellencamp. Bloomington: Indiana University Press, 1990.

———. "Temporality, Storage, Legibility: Freud, Marey, and the Cinema." *Critical Inquiry* 22, no. 2 (winter 1996): 313–43.

———. "The Voice in the Cinema: The Articulation of Body and Space." In *Narrative, Apparatus, Ideology*. Ed. by Philip Rosen. New York: Columbia University Press, 1986.

Doherty, Thomas. *Pre-Code Hollywood: Sex, Immorality and Insurrection in American Cinema, 1930–1934*. New York: Columbia University Press, 1999.

———. *Projections of War: Hollywood, American Culture, and World War II*. New York: Columbia University Press, 1993.

Douglas, Mary. *Purity and Danger: An Analysis of Concepts of Pollution and Taboo*. 1966. New York: Routledge, 2002.

Douglas, Susan. *Inventing American Broadcasting, 1899–1922*. Baltimore: Johns Hopkins University Press, 1987.

Draper, Ellen. "'Controversy Has Probably Destroyed Forever the Context':

The Miracle and Movie Censorship in America in the 1950s." In *Controlling Hollywood: Censorship and Regulation in the Studio Era*. Ed. by Matthew Bernstein. New Brunswick: Rutgers University Press, 1999.

Duffy, John. *The Sanitarians: A History of American Public Health*. Urbana: University of Illinois Press, 1990.

Dyer, Richard. *Stars*. London: BFI, 1979.

———. "White." *Screen* 29, no. 4 (1988): 44–65.

———. *White*. New York: Routledge, 1997.

Dysinger, W. S., and Christian A. Ruckmick. *The Emotional Responses of Children to the Motion Picture Situation*. New York: Macmillan, 1933.

Eagleton, Terry. *Criticism and Ideology*. London: Verso, 1978.

Eberwein, Robert. *Sex Ed: Film, Video, and the Framework of Desire*. New Brunswick: Rutgers University Press, 1999.

Eco, Umberto. *Travels in Hyperreality: Essays*. San Diego: Harcourt, 1986.

Elliott, Godfrey M. *Film and Education: A Symposium on the Role of the Film in the Field of Education*. New York: Philosophical Library, 1948.

Elsaesser, Thomas. "Primary Identification and the Historical Subject: Fassbinder and Germany." In *Narrative, Apparatus, Ideology*. Ed. by Philip Rosen. New York: Columbia University Press, 1986.

———, ed. *Early Cinema: Space, Frame, Narrative*. London: BFI, 1990.

Eng, David. *Racial Castration: Managing Masculinity in Asian America*. Durham: Duke University Press, 2001.

Ernst, Morris L., and Pare Lorentz. *Censored: The Private Life of the Movie*. New York: Jonathan Cape, 1930.

Essex-Lopresti, Michael. "The Medical Film 1897–1997, Part I: The First Half-Century." *Journal of Audiovisual Media in Medicine* 21, no. 1 (1998): 7–12.

Etheridge, Elizabeth W. *Sentinel for Health: A History of the Centers for Disease Control*. Berkeley: University of California Press, 1992.

Ewald, Paul. *Plague Time: How Stealth Infections Cause Cancers, Heart Disease, and Other Deadly Ailments*. New York: Free Press, 2000.

Ewen, Elizabeth. *Immigrant Women in the Land of Dollars: Life and Culture on the Lower East Side, 1890–1925*. New York: Monthly Review, 1985.

Ewen, Stuart. *Captains of Consciousness: Advertising and the Social Roots of the Consumer Culture*. New York: McGraw-Hill, 1977.

Ewen, Stuart, and Elizabeth Ewen. *Channels of Desire: Mass Images and the Shaping of American Consciousness.* Minneapolis: University of Minnesota Press, 1992.

Facey, Paul W. *The Legion of Decency: A Sociological Analysis of the Emergence and Development of a Social Pressure Group.* 1945. New York: Arno, 1974.

Fearing, Franklin. "Influence of Movies on Attitudes and Behavior." *Annals of the American Academy of Political and Social Science* 254 (1947): 70–79.

Fell, John, ed. *Film Before Griffith.* Berkeley: University of California Press, 1983.

Fenster, Mark. *Conspiracy Theories: Secrecy and Power in American Culture.* Minneapolis: University of Minnesota Press, 1999.

Fern, George H. *Teaching with Films.* Milwaukee: Bruce Publishing, 1946.

Feuer, Jane. "The Concept of Live Television: Ontology as Ideology." In *Regarding Television: Critical Approaches.* Ed. by E. Ann Kaplan. Los Angeles: AFI, 1983.

Film Evaluation Board of the Advisory Board on Education and Division of Mathematics. *The Use of Films and Television in Mathematics Education.* Washington: National Academy of Sciences/National Research Council. Publication no. 567, 1957.

Flaherty, Robert. "The Belcher Islands of Hudson Bay: Their Discovery and Exploration." *Geographical Review* 5, no. 6 (June 1918): 433–43.

Forman, Henry James. *Our Movie Made Children.* New York: Macmillan, 1933.

Foucault, Michel. *The Birth of the Clinic: An Archaeology of Medical Perception.* New York: Random House, 1973.

———. *Discipline and Punish: The Birth of the Prison.* New York: Random House, 1977.

———. *The History of Sexuality, Volume I: An Introduction.* New York: Random House, 1978.

———. *The Order of Things: An Archaeology of the Human Sciences.* New York: Random House, 1973.

Fox, Richard Wightman, and T. J. Jackson Lears, eds. *The Culture of Consumption: Critical Essays in American History, 1880–1980.* New York: Pantheon, 1983.

Friedman, James, ed. *Reality Squared: Televisual Discourse on the Real*. New Brunswick: Rutgers University Press, 2002.

Furman, Bess. *A Profile of the United States Public Health Service, 1798–1948*. Washington: u.s. Dept. of Health, Education and Welfare, 1973.

Furniss, Maureen. *Art in Motion: Animation Aesthetics*. Sydney, Australia: John Libbey, 1998.

Gabaccia, Donna. *Immigration and American Diversity: A Social and Cultural History*. Oxford: Blackwell, 2001.

Garber, Marjorie, Jann Matlock, and Rebecca Walkowitz, eds. *Media Spectacles*. New York: Routledge, 1993.

Garrett, Laurie. *The Coming Plague: Newly Emerging Diseases in a World Out of Balance*. New York: Penguin, 1994.

Gibson, James J. ed. *Motion Picture Testing and Research*. Washington: US Gov't. Printing Office, 1947.

Gilman, Sander. *Difference and Pathology*. Ithaca: Cornell University Press, 1985.

———. *Picturing Health and Illness: Images of Identity and Difference*. Baltimore: Johns Hopkins University Press, 1995.

Ginzberg, Lori. *Women and the Work of Benevolence: Morality, Politics, and Class in the Nineteenth-Century United States*. New Haven: Yale University Press, 1990.

Gipson, Henry Clay. *Films in Business and Industry*. New York: McGraw-Hill, 1947.

Gitlin, Todd. *The Whole World Is Watching: Mass Media in the Making and Unmaking of the New Left*. Berkeley: University of California Press, 1980.

Gledhill, Christine, ed. *Stardom: Industry of Desire*. New York: Routledge, 1991.

Goldfarb, Brian. *Visual Pedagogy: Media Cultures in and Beyond the Classroom*. Durham: Duke University Press, 2002.

Gomery, Douglas. *Shared Pleasures: A History of Movie Presentation in the United States*. Madison: University of Wisconsin Press, 1992.

Gould, Tony. *A Summer Plague: Polio and Its Survivors*. New Haven: Yale University Press, 1995.

Guerrero, Ed. *Framing Blackness: The African American Image in Film*. Philadelphia: Temple University Press, 1993.

Guillemin, Jeanne. *Anthrax: The Investigation of a Deadly Outbreak*. Berkeley: University of California Press, 1999.

Gunning, Tom. "An Aesthetic of Astonishment: Early Film and the (In)Credulous Spectator." *Art and Text* 34 (spring 1989): 31–45.

———. "The Cinema of Attractions: Early Film, Its Spectator, and the Avant-Garde." In *Early Cinema: Space, Frame, and Narrative*. Ed. by Thomas Elsaesser. London: British Film Institute, 1990.

———. "Tracing the Individual Body: Photography, Detectives, and Early Cinema." In *Cinema and the Invention of Modern Life*. Ed. by Leo Charney and Vanessa R. Schwartz. Berkeley: University of California Press, 1995.

Haas, Kenneth B. and Harry Q. Packer. *Preparation and Use of Visual Aids*. New York: Prentice, 1946.

Hammonds, Evelynn. "Race, Sex, AIDS: The Construction of 'Other.' " *Radical America* 20.6: 28–37.

Handel, Leo. *Hollywood Looks at Its Audience: A Report of Film Audience Research*. Urbana: University of Illinois Press, 1950.

Hansen, Miriam. *Babel and Babylon. Spectatorship in American Silent Film*. Cambridge: Harvard University Press, 1991.

Haraway, Donna. *Simians, Cyborgs and Women: The Reinvention of Nature*. New York: Routledge, 1991.

Harden, Victoria A. *Inventing the NIH: Federal Biomedical Research Policy, 1887–1937*. Baltimore: Johns Hopkins University Press, 1986.

Hardy, Phil. *Science Fiction*. The Overlook Film Encyclopedia Series. 3rd ed. Woodstock, New York: Overlook, 1995.

Harpold, Terry. "Dark Continents: A Critique of Internet Metageographies." *Postmodern Culture* 9, no. 2 (1999): 5. At http://muse.jhu.edu/journals/postmodern_culture/.

Hart, Kylo-Patrick R. *The AIDS Movie: Representing a Pandemic in Film and Television*. New York: Haworth, 2000.

Hays, J. N. *The Burdens of Disease: Epidemics and Human Response in Western History*. New Brunswick: Rutgers University Press, 1998.

Hendershot, Cyndy. *Paranoia, the Bomb, and 1950s Science Fiction Films*. Bowling Green: Bowling Green State University Popular Press, 1999.

Henriksen, Margot A. *Dr. Strangelove's America: Society and Culture in the Atomic Age*. Berkeley: University of California Press, 1997.

Hill, Mike, ed. *Whiteness: A Critical Reader*. New York: New York University Press, 1997.

Hillis, Ken. *Digital Sensations: Space, Identity, and Embodiment in Virtual Reality*. Minneapolis: University of Minnesota Press, 1999.

Hills, Jill. *The Struggle for Control of Global Communication: The Formative Century*. Urbana: University of Illinois Press, 2002.

Hoban, Charles F. *Movies That Teach*. New York: Dryden, 1946.

Hobsbawm, Eric. *Nations and Nationalism Since 1780: Programme, Myth, Reality*. New York: Cambridge University Press, 1990.

Hoerder, Dirk. *Cultures in Contact: World Migrations in the Second Millennium*. Durham: Duke University Press, 2002.

Hofstadter, Richard. *The Paranoid Style in American Politics and Other Essays*. New York: Knopf, 1965.

Holaday, P. W. *Getting Ideas From the Movies*. New York: Macmillan, 1933.

Huettig, Mae D. *Economic Control of the Motion Picture Industry: A Study in Industrial Organization*. Philadelphia: University of Pennsylvania Press, 1944.

Huyssen, Andreas. "Mass Culture as Woman: Modernism's Other." In *Studies in Entertainment: Critical Approaches to Mass Culture*. Ed. by Tania Modleski. Bloomington: Indiana University Press, 1986.

Isenberg, Michael T. *War on Film: The American Cinema and World War I, 1914–1941*. Rutherford, N.J.: Associated University Press, 1981.

Jacobs, Lea. "Reformers and Spectators: The Film Education Movement in the Thirties." *Camera Obscura* 22 (1990).

———. *The Wages of Sin: Censorship and the Fallen Woman Film, 1928–1942*. Madison: University of Wisconsin Press, 1991.

Jacobs, Lewis. *The Rise of the American Film: A Critical History*. New York: Harcourt, 1939.

Jacobson, Matthew Frye. *Whiteness of a Different Color: European Immigrants and the Alchemy of Race*. Cambridge, Mass.: Harvard University Press, 1998.

Jacobus, Mary, Evelyn Fox-Keller, and Sally Shuttleworth, eds. *Body/Politics: Women and the Discourses of Science*. New York: Routledge, 1990.

Jameson, Fredric. *The Geopolitical Aesthetic: Cinema and Space in the World System*. Bloomington: Indiana University Press, 1992.

Jameson, Fredric. *Postmodernism, or, the Cultural Logic of Late Capitalism.* Durham: Duke University Press, 1991.

Jameson, Fredric, and Masao Miyoshi, eds. *The Cultures of Globalization.* Durham: Duke University Press, 1998.

Jarvie, Ian. *Hollywood's Overseas Campaign: The North Atlantic Movie Trade, 1920–1950.* New York: Cambridge University Press, 1992.

Jowett, Garth. " 'A Significant Medium for the Communication of Ideas': The *Miracle* Decision and the Decline of Motion Picture Censorship, 1952–1968." In *Movie Censorship and American Culture.* Ed. by Francis G. Couvares. Washington: Smithsonian, 1996.

———. *Film: The Democratic Art.* Boston: Little, Brown, 1976.

Jowett, Garth, Ian C. Jarvie, and Kathryn H. Fuller. *Children and the Movies: Media Influence and the Payne Fund Controversy.* New York: Cambridge University Press, 1996.

Jowett, Garth, Penny Reath, and Monica Schouten. "The Control of Mass Entertainment Media in Canada, the United States and Great Britain: Historical Surveys." In *Report of the Royal Commission on Violence in the Communications Industry* 4. Toronto: Queen's, 1977.

Joyrich, Lynne. *Re-Viewing Reception: Television, Gender, and Postmodern Culture.* Bloomington: Indiana University Press, 1996.

Juhasz, Alexandra. AIDS TV: *Identity, Community, and Alternative Video.* Durham: Duke University Press, 1995.

Kaplan, E. Ann, ed. *Psychoanalysis and Cinema.* New York: Routledge, 1990.

Karlen, Arno. *Biography of a Germ.* New York: Pantheon, 2000.

Karpf, Anne. *Doctoring the Media: The Reporting of Health and Medicine.* London: Routledge, 1988.

Kevles, Bettyann Holtzmann. *Naked to the Bone: Medical Imaging in the Twentieth Century.* New Brunswick: Rutgers University Press, 1997.

King, Geoff. *Mapping Reality: An Exploration of Cultural Cartographies.* New York: St. Martin's, 1996.

King, Stephen. "Danse Macabre." In *Invasion of the Body Snatchers.* Ed. by Al LaValley. New Brunswick: Rutgers University Press, 1989.

Kinsella, James. *Covering the Plague:* AIDS *and the American Media.* New Brunswick: Rutgers University Press, 1989.

Kinsey, Alfred C., and Institute for Sex Research. *Sexual Behavior in the Human Female*. Philadelphia: W. B. Saunders, 1953.

———. *Sexual Behavior in the Human Male*. Philadelphia: W. B. Saunders, 1948.

Kirby, Lynne. *Parallel Tracks: The Railroad and Silent Cinema*. Durham: Duke University Press, 1997.

Knee, Adam. *The American Science Fiction Film and Fifties Culture*. Ph.D. diss., New York University, 1997.

Kolata, Gina. *Flu: The Story of the Great Influenza Pandemic of 1918 and the Search for the Virus That Caused It*. New York: Simon and Schuster, 1999.

Kolko, Beth E., Lisa Nakamura, and Gilbert B. Rodman, eds. *Race in Cyberspace*. New York: Routledge, 2000.

Koppes, Clayton R., and Gregory D. Black. *Hollywood Goes to War: How Politics, Profits, and Propaganda Shaped World War II Movies*. New York: Macmillan, 1987.

Kraut, Alan M. *Silent Travelers: Germs, Genes, and the "Immigrant Menace."* New York: Basic Books, 1994.

Kroker, Arthur, and Marilouise Kroker. *Body Invaders: Panic Sex in America*. New York: St. Martin's, 1987.

Kuhn, Annette, ed. *Alien Zone: Cultural Theory and Contemporary Science Fiction Cinema*. New York: Verso, 1990.

———. *Cinema, Censorship and Sexuality, 1909–1925*. New York: Routledge, 1988.

Lacan, Jacques. *Écrits*. 1958. New York: Norton, 1977.

Laine, Elizabeth. *Motion Pictures and Radio: Modern Techniques for Education*. New York: McGraw-Hill, 1938.

Latour, Bruno. *Science in Action: How to Follow Scientists and Engineers Through Society*. Philadelphia: Open University Press, 1987.

LaValley, Al, ed. *Invasion of the Body Snatchers, Don Siegel, director*. New Brunswick: Rutgers University Press, 1989.

Lee, Kelley. *Historical Dictionary of the World Health Organization*. London: Scarecrow, 1998.

Lee, Robert G. *Orientals: Asian Americans in Popular Culture*. Philadelphia: Temple University Press, 1999.

Lefebvre, Henri. *The Production of Space*. Trans. Donald Nicholson-Smith. Cambridge: Blackwell, 1991.

Legion of Decency. *Motion Pictures Classified by National Legion of Decency*. New York: National Legion of Decency, 1948.

Lemonick, Michael D. "Return to the Hot Zone." *Time*, May 22 (1995): 63.

Lentz, Kirsten Marthe. "*Quality* versus *Relevance*: Feminism, Race, and the Politics of the Sign in 1970s Television." *Camera Obscura* 43, no. 15 (2000): 45–93.

Lev, Peter. *American Films of the '70s: Conflicting Visions*. Austin: University of Texas Press, 2000.

Link, Arthur, and Richard L. McCormick. *Progressivism*. Arlington Heights, Ill.: Harlan Davidson, 1983.

Lowery, Shearon, and Melvin De Fleur. *Milestones in Mass Communications Research*. 2nd ed. New York: Longman, 1988.

Lucanio, Patrick. *Them or Us: Archetypal Interpretations of Fifties Alien Invasion Films*. Bloomington: Indiana University Press, 1987.

Lundell, Allan. *Virus! The Secret World of Computer Invaders that Breed and Destroy*. Chicago: Contemporary, 1989.

MacCabe, Colin. "Realism and the Cinema: Notes on Some Brechtian Theses." *Screen* 15, no. 2 (1974).

MacCann, Richard Dyer. *The People's Films: A Political History of u.s. Government Motion Pictures*. New York: Hastings, 1973.

Manovich, Lev. "The Paradoxes of Digital Photography." In *Photography After Photography*. Exhibition Catalog. Germany, 1995.

Marchand, Roland. *Advertising the American Dream: Making Way for Modernity, 1920–1940*. Berkeley: University of California Press, 1985.

Marchetti, Gina. *Romance and the Yellow Peril: Race, Sex, and Discursive Strategies in Hollywood Fiction*. Berkeley: University of California Press, 1993.

Mattelart, Armand. *Mapping World Communication: War, Progress, Culture*. Trans. Susan Emanuel and James A. Cohen. Minneapolis: University of Minnesota Press, 1994.

———. *Networking the World, 1794–2000*. Trans. Liz Carey-Libbrecht and James A. Cohen. Minneapolis: University of Minnesota Press, 2000.

May, Elaine Tyler. *Homeward Bound: American Families in the Cold War Era*. New York: Harper Collins, 1988.

May, Mark A., and Arthur A. Lumsdaine. *Learning from Films.* New Haven: Yale University Press, 1958.

McCarthy, Todd, and Charles Flynn, eds. *Kings of the B's: Working Within the Hollywood System. An Anthology of Film History and Criticism.* New York: E. P. Dutton, 1975.

McClintock, Anne. *Imperial Leather: Race, Gender and Sexuality in the Colonial Contest.* New York: Routledge, 1995.

McCormick, Joseph B. *Level 4: Virus Hunters of the CDC.* Atlanta: Turner, 1996.

McLuhan, Marshall. *Understanding Media: The Extensions of Man.* 1964. Cambridge: MIT Press, 1994.

Means, Richard K. *A History of Health Education in the United States.* Philadelphia: Lea and Febiger, 1962.

Melley, Timothy. *Empire of Conspiracy: The Culture of Paranoia in Postwar America.* Ithaca: Cornell University Press, 2000.

Meyerowitz, Joanne, ed. *Not June Cleaver: Women and Gender in Postwar America, 1945–1960.* Philadelphia: Temple University Press, 1994.

Miller, D. A. "Anal Rope." *Inside/Out: Lesbian Theories, Gay Theories.* Ed. by Diana Fuss. New York: Routledge, 1991.

Miller, Stephen Paul. *The Seventies Now: Culture as Surveillance.* Durham: Duke University Press, 1999.

Mock, James R., and Cedric Larson, *Words That Won the War: The Story of the Committee on Public Information, 1917–1919.* Princeton: Princeton University Press, 1939.

Moley, Raymond. *Are We Movie-Made?* New York: Macy-Masius, 1938.

———. *The Hays Office.* New York: Bobbs-Merrill, 1945.

Monmonier, Mark. *How to Lie with Maps.* Chicago: University of Chicago Press, 1991.

Morse, Margaret. "An Ontology of Everyday Distraction: The Freeway, the Mall, and Television." In *Logics of Television: Essays in Cultural Criticism.* Ed. by Patricia Mellencamp. Bloomington: Indiana University Press, 1990.

———. "The Television News Personality and Credibility: Reflections on the News in Transition." In *Studies in Entertainment: Critical Approaches to Mass Culture.* Ed. by Tania Modleski. Bloomington: Indiana University Press, 1986.

Morse, Margaret. *Virtualities: Television, Media Art, and Cyberculture.* Bloomington: Indiana University Press, 1998.

Mould, David H. *American Newsfilm, 1914–1919: The Underexposed War.* New York: Garland, 1983.

Mullan, Fitzhugh. *Plagues and Politics: The Story of the United States Public Health Service.* New York: Basic Books, 1989.

Mulvey, Laura. "Visual Pleasure and Narrative Cinema." In *Narrative, Apparatus, Ideology.* Ed. by Philip Rosen. New York: Columbia University Press, 1986.

Musser, Charles. *Before the Nickelodeon: Edwin S. Porter and the Edison Manufacturing Company.* Berkeley: University of California Press, 1991.

———. *The Emergence of Cinema: The American Screen to 1907.* New York: Scribner's, 1990.

Musser, Charles, and Carol Nelson. *High-Class Moving Pictures: Lyman H. Howe and the Forgotten Era of Traveling Exhibition, 1880–1920.* Princeton: Princeton University Press, 1991.

Neale, Steve. "Masculinity as Spectacle: Reflections on Men and Mainstream Cinema." In *Screening the Male: Exploring Masculinities in Hollywood Cinema.* Ed. by Steven Cohan and Ina Rae Hark. New York: Routledge, 1993.

Nelson, Henry B. *Mass Media and Education.* Chicago: University of Chicago Press, 1954.

Nichols, Bill. *Representing Reality: Issues and Concepts in Documentary.* Bloomington: Indiana University Press, 1991.

Nichtenhauser, Adolf. "A History of Motion Pictures in Medicine." Bethesda: National Library of Medicine, History of Medicine Division, c. 1950. MS. c. 380, boxes 1 and 2.

O'Connor, John E., and Martin A. Jackson, eds. *American History/American Film: Interpreting the Hollywood Image.* New York: Frederick Ungar, 1979.

O'Donnell, Patrick. "Engendering Paranoia in Contemporary Narrative." *boundary 2* 19, no. 1 (1992): 181–204.

Oldstone, Michael. *Viruses, Plagues, and History.* New York: Oxford University Press, 1998.

Omi, Michael, and Howard Winant. *Racial Formation in the United States: From the 1960s to the 1990s.* New York: Routledge, 1994.

Orvell, Miles. *The Real Thing: Imitation and Authenticity in American Culture, 1880–1940*. Chapel Hill: University of North Carolina Press, 1989.

Packard, Vance. *The Hidden Persuaders*. New York: D. McKay, 1957.

Parascondola, John. "VD at the Movies: PHS Films of the 1930s and 1940s." *Public Health Reports* 3 (March/April 1996): 173–75.

Parker, Andrew, Mary Russo, Doris Sommer, and Patricia Yeager, eds. *Nationalisms and Sexualities*. New York: Routledge, 1992.

Patton, Cindy. *Fatal Advice: How Safe-Sex Education Went Wrong*. Durham: Duke University Press, 1996.

———. *Inventing AIDS*. New York: Routledge, 1990.

———. *Sex and Germs: The Politics of AIDS*. New York: Black Rose, 1986.

Peary, Danny. *Cult Movies: A Hundred Ways to Find the Reel Thing*. London: Vermilion, 1982.

Peirce, Charles Sanders. "What Is a Sign?" In *The Essential Peirce: Selected Philosophical Writings, vol. 2 (1893–1913)*. Peirce Edition Project. Bloomington: Indiana University Press, 1998.

Peiss, Kathy. *Cheap Amusements: Working Women and Leisure in Turn-of-the-Century New York*. Philadelphia: Temple University Press, 1986.

Penley, Constance, Elisabeth Lyon, Lynn Spigel, and Janet Bergstrom, eds. *Close Encounters: Film, Feminism, and Science Fiction*. Minneapolis: University of Minnesota Press, 1991.

Penley, Constance, and Sharon Willis, eds. *Male Trouble*. Minneapolis: University of Minnesota Press, 1993.

Perlman, William J., ed. *The Movies on Trial*. New York: Macmillan, 1936.

Pernick, Martin. *The Black Stork: Eugenics and the Death of "Defective" Babies in American Medicine and Motion Pictures Since 1915*. New York: Oxford University Press, 1996.

———. "Sex Education Films, U.S. Government, 1920s." *Isis* 84, no. 4 (1993): 766–68.

Peters, Charles C. *Motion Pictures and Standards of Morality*. New York: Macmillan, 1933.

Peterson, Ruth C., and L. L. Thurstone. *Motion Pictures and the Social Attitudes of Children*. New York: Macmillan, 1933.

Pilling, Jayne, ed. *A Reader in Animation Studies*. Sydney, Australia: John Libbey, 1997.

Polan, Dana. *Power and Paranoia: History, Narrative, and the American Cin-ema, 1940–1950*. New York: Columbia University Press, 1986.

Preston, Richard. "Crisis in the Hot Zone." *New Yorker* October 26, 1992, 58–81.

———. *The Hot Zone*. New York: Doubleday, 1994.

Puar, Jasbir K., and Amit S. Rai. "Monster, Terrorist, Fag: The War on Ter-rorism and the Production of Docile Patriots." *Social Text* 72 (fall 2002): 117–48.

Quart, Leonard, and Albert Auster. *American Film and Society since 1945*. 2nd ed. New York: Praeger, 1991.

Rabinovitz, Lauren. *For the Love of Pleasure: Women, Movies, and Culture in Turn-of-the-Century Chicago*. New Brunswick: Rutgers University Press, 1998.

Raimondo, Meredith. "The Next Wave: Media Maps of the 'Spread of AIDS.'" Ph.D. diss., Emory University, 1999.

Regis, Ed. *Virus Ground Zero: Stalking the Killer Viruses with the Centers for Disease Control*. New York: Simon and Schuster, 1996.

Renov, Michael, ed. *Theorizing Documentary*. New York: Routledge, 1993.

Renshaw, Samuel. *Children's Sleep*. New York: Macmillan, 1933.

Riesman, David, Revel Denney, and Nathan Glazer. *The Lonely Crowd: A Study of the Changing American Character*. New Haven: Yale University Press, 1952.

Robbins, Bruce, ed. *The Phantom Public Sphere*. Minneapolis: University of Minnesota Press, 1993.

Rodowick, David N. "Madness, Authority and Ideology: The Domestic Melo-drama of the 1950s." In *Home Is Where the Heart Is: Studies in Melodrama and the Woman's Film*. Ed. by Christine Gledhill. London: BFI, 1987.

Roediger, David R. *The Wages of Whiteness: Race and the Making of the Ameri-can Working Class*. New York: Verso, 1999.

Rogin, Michael. *Ronald Reagan, the Movie and Other Episodes in Political De-monology*. Berkeley: University of California Press, 1987.

Rony, Fatimah Tobing. *The Third Eye: Race, Cinema, and Ethnographic Spec-tacle*. Durham: Duke University Press, 1996.

Rosen, George. *A History of Public Health*. New York: MD Publications, 1958.

Rosen, Philip. "Document and Documentary: On the Persistence of Historical Concepts." In *Theorizing Documentary*. Ed. by Michael Renov. New York: Routledge, 1993.

———, ed. *Narrative, Apparatus, Ideology*. New York: Columbia University Press, 1986.

———. "Old and New: Image, Indexicality and Historicity in the Digital Utopia." *Iconics* 4 (1998): 1–45.

Ross, Andrew. "Hacking Away at the Counterculture." In *Electronic Media and Technoculture*. Ed. by John Thornton Caldwell. New Brunswick: Rutgers University Press, 2000.

Rubin, Gayle. "Thinking Sex: Notes for a Radical Theory of the Politics of Sexuality." In *Pleasure and Danger: Exploring Female Sexuality*. Ed. by Carole S. Vance. Boston: Routledge, 1984.

Ryan, Frank. *Virus X: Tracking the New Killer Plagues: Out of the Present and Into the Future*. Boston: Little, Brown, 1997.

Ryan, Michael, and Douglas Kellner. *Camera Politica: The Politics and Ideology of Contemporary Hollywood Film*. Bloomington: Indiana University Press, 1988.

Samuels, Stuart. "The Age of Conspiracy and Conformity: Invasion of the Body Snatchers." In *American History/American Film: Interpreting the American Image*. Ed. by John O'Connor and Martin A. Jackson. New York: Frederick Ungar, 1979.

Sayre, Nora. *Running Time: Films of the Cold War*. New York: Dial, 1982.

Schaefer, Eric. *"Bold! Daring! Shocking! True!" A History of Exploitation Films, 1910–1959*. Durham: Duke University Press, 1999.

Schivelbusch, Wolfgang. *The Railway Journey: The Industrialization of Time and Space in the 19th Century*. Berkeley: University of California Press, 1977.

Scott, Joan Wallach. *Gender and the Politics of History*. New York: Columbia University Press, 1988.

Sedgwick, Eve Kosofsky. *Between Men: English Literature and Male Homosocial Desire*. New York: Columbia University Press, 1985.

———. *Epistemology of the Closet*. Berkeley: University of California Press, 1990.

Seed, David. *American Science Fiction and the Cold War: Literature and Film*. Chicago: Fitzroy Dearborn, 1999.

Segrave, Kerry. *American Films Abroad: Hollywood's Domination of the World's Movie Screens*. Jefferson, N.C.: McFarland, 1997.

Sekula, Allan. "The Body and the Archive." *October* 39 (winter 1986): 3–64.

Shah, Nayan. *Contagious Divides: Epidemics and Race in San Francisco's Chinatown*. Berkeley: University of California Press, 2001.

Sharett, Christopher, ed. *Crisis Cinema: The Apocalyptic Idea in Postmodern Narrative Film*. Washington: Maisonneuve, 1993.

Shilts, Randy. *And the Band Played On: Politics, People, and the AIDS Epidemic*. New York: St. Martin's, 1987.

Shorter, Edward. *The Health Century*. New York: Doubleday, 1987.

Shuttleworth, Frank K., and Mark A. May. *The Social Conduct and Attitudes of Movie Fans*. New York: Macmillan, 1933.

Siddiqi, Javed. *World Health and World Politics: The World Health Organization and the UN System*. Columbia: University of South Carolina Press, 1995.

Silverman, Kaja. "Historical Trauma and Male Subjectivity." In *Psychoanalysis and Cinema*. Ed. by E. Ann Kaplan. New York: Routledge, 1990.

Simpson, James B., comp. *Simpson's Contemporary Quotations*. Boston: Houghton Mifflin, 1988.

Sklar, Robert. *Movie-Made America*. New York: Random House, 1975.

Sloan, Kay. *The Loud Silents: Origins of the Social Problem Film*. Chicago: University of Illinois Press, 1988.

Smith, Ken. *Mental Hygiene: Classroom Films, 1945–1970*. New York: Blast, 1999.

Smith-Rosenberg, Caroll. *Disorderly Conduct: Visions of Gender in Victorian America*. New York: Oxford University Press, 1985.

Smoodin, Eric. *Animating Culture: Hollywood Cartoons from the Sound Era*. New Brunswick: Rutgers University Press, 1993.

Smulyan, Susan. *Selling Radio: The Commercialization of American Broadcasting, 1920–1934*. Washington: Smithsonian, 1994.

Snead, James. *White Screens, Black Images: Hollywood from the Dark Side*. New York: Routledge, 1994.

Snyder, Robert L. *Pare Lorentz and the Documentary Film*. Norman: University of Oklahoma Press, 1968.

Sobchack, Vivian. *Screening Space: The American Science Fiction Film*. 2nd ed. New Brunswick: Rutgers University Press, 1987.

————. "The Virginity of Astronauts: Sex and the Science Fiction Film." In *Shadows of the Magic Lamp: Fantasy and Science Fiction in Film*. Ed. by George Slusser and Eric S. Rabkin. Carbondale: Southern Illinois University Press, 1985.

Sontag, Susan. *Against Interpretation, and Other Essays*. New York: Farrar, Straus and Giroux, 1966.

————. *Illness as Metaphor and AIDS and Its Metaphors*. 1977. New York: Doubleday, 1989.

Spigel, Lynn. *Make Room for TV: Television and the Family Ideal in Postwar America*. Chicago: University of Chicago Press, 1992.

Springer, Claudia. *Electronic Eros: Bodies and Desire in the Postindustrial Age*. Austin: University of Texas Press, 1996.

Staiger, Janet. *Interpreting Films: Studies in the Historical Reception of American Films*. Princeton: Princeton University Press, 1992.

Stam, Robert. "Television News and Its Spectator." In *Regarding Television: Critical Approaches*. Ed. by E. Ann Kaplan. Los Angeles: AFI, 1983.

Stam, Robert, Robert Burgoyne, and Sandy Flitterman-Lewis. *New Vocabularies in Film Semiotics: Structuralism, Post-Structuralism and Beyond*. New York: Routledge, 1992.

Starr, Paul. *The Social Transformation of American Medicine*. New York: Basic Books, 1982.

Steffen-Fluhr, Nancy. "Women and the Inner Game of Don Siegel's *Invasion of the Body Snatchers*." *Science Fiction Studies* 11, no. 2 (July 1984): 139–53.

Suid, Lawrence H., ed. *Film and Propaganda in America: A Documentary History. Volume IV: 1945 and After*. New York: Greenwood, 1991.

Sze, Szeming. *The Origins of The World Health Organization: A Personal Memoir, 1945–1948*. Boca Raton: LISZ Publications, 1982.

Tarratt, Margaret. "Monsters from the Id." In *Film Genre Reader II*. Ed. by Barry Keith Grant. Austin: University of Texas Press, 1995.

Telotte, J. P. *Replications: A Robotic History of the Science Fiction Film*. Urbana: University of Illinois Press, 1995.

Thompson, Kristin. *Exporting Entertainment: America in the World Film Market, 1907–1934*. London: BFI, 1985.

Thompson, Kristin, and David Bordwell. *Film History: An Introduction*. 2nd ed. New York: McGraw-Hill, 2003.

Thrower, Norman J. W. *Maps and Civilization: Cartography in Culture and Society*. 1972. Chicago: University of Chicago Press, 1996.

Tomes, Nancy. *The Gospel of Germs: Men, Women, and the Microbe in American Life*. Cambridge: Harvard University Press, 1998.

Treichler, Paula. "AIDS, Africa, and Cultural Theory." *Transition* 51 (1991).

———. "AIDS Narrative on Television." In *Writing AIDS: Gay Literature, Language, and Analysis*. Ed. by Timothy Murphy and Suzanne Poirier. New York: Columbia University Press, 1993.

———. *How to Have Theory in an Epidemic: Cultural Chronicles of AIDS*. Durham: Duke University Press, 1999.

Treichler, Paula, Lisa Cartwright, and Constance Penley, eds. *The Visible Woman: Imaging Technologies, Gender, and Science*. New York: New York University Press, 1998.

Turkle, Sherry. *Life on the Screen: Identity in the Age of the Internet*. New York: Simon and Schuster, 1995.

Vasey, Ruth. "Beyond Sex and Violence: 'Industry Policy' and the Regulation of Hollywood Movies, 1922–1939." *Controlling Hollywood: Censorship and Regulation in the Studio Era*. Ed. by Matthew Bernstein. New Brunswick: Rutgers University Press, 1999.

———. *The World According to Hollywood, 1918–1939*. Madison: University of Wisconsin Press, 1997.

Wald, Priscilla, Nancy Tomes, and Lisa Lynch, eds. *American Literary History* 14, no. 4 (2002).

Walsh, Frank. *Sin and Censorship: The Catholic Church and the Motion Picture Industry*. New Haven: Yale University Press, 1996.

Ward, Larry Wayne. *The Motion Picture Goes to War: The U.S. Government Film Effort during World War I*. 1981. Ann Arbor: University of Michigan Research Press, 1985.

Warren, Bill. *Keep Watching the Skies! American Science Fiction Movies of the Fifties. Volume I, 1950–1957*. Jefferson, N.C.: McFarland, 1982.

Watney, Simon. "Missionary Positions." *Critical Quarterly* 30 (1989).

———. *Policing Desire: AIDS, Pornography, and the Media*. Minneapolis: University of Minnesota Press, 1987.

Watson, Mary Ann. *The Expanding Vista: American Television in the Kennedy Years*. Durham: Duke University Press, 1994.

Weart, Spencer R. *Nuclear Fear: A History of Images*. Cambridge, Mass.: Harvard University Press, 1988.

Weeks, Jeffrey. *Sex, Politics, and Society: The Regulation of Sexuality Since 1800*. New York: Longman, 1989.

Weis, Elisabeth, and John Belton, eds. *Film Sound: Theory and Practice*. New York: Columbia University Press, 1985.

Weisse, Allen B. *Medical Odysseys: The Different and Sometimes Unexpected Pathways to Twentieth-Century Medical Discoveries*. New Brunswick: Rutgers University Press, 1991.

Whalen, David Joseph. *The Origins of Satellite Communications, 1945–1965*. Washington: Smithsonian, 2002.

White, Suzanne M. "*Mom and Dad* (1944): Venereal Disease Exploitation." *Bulletin of the History of Medicine* 62 (1988): 252–70.

Wiebe, Robert H. *The Search for Order, 1877–1920*. New York: Hill, 1967.

Willemen, Paul. "The Third Cinema Question: Notes and Reflections." In *Questions of Third Cinema*. Ed. by Jim Pines and Paul Willemen. London: BFI, 1989.

Williams, Juan. *Eyes on the Prize: America's Civil Rights Years, 1954–1965*. New York: Viking, 1987.

Williams, Linda. "Film Bodies: Gender, Genre, and Excess." In *Film Genre Reader II*. Ed. by Barry K. Grant. Austin: University of Texas Press, 1995.

———. "Film Body: An Implantation of Perversions." In *Narrative, Apparatus, Ideology*. Ed. by Philip Rosen. New York: Columbia University Press, 1986.

———. *Hard Core: Power, Pleasure, and the "Frenzy of the Visible."* Berkeley: University of California Press, 1989.

Williams, Ralph Chester. *The United States Public Health Service, 1798–1950*. Richmond: Whittet and Shepperson, 1951.

Williams, Raymond. *Television: Technology and Cultural Form*. Glasgow: Fontana/Collins, 1974.

Wilson, Sloan. *The Man in the Gray Flannel Suit*. New York: Simon and Schuster, 1955.

Winston, Brian. *Claiming the Real: The Documentary Film Revisited*. London: BFI, 1995.

Winston, Brian. *Technologies of Seeing: Photography, Cinematography and Tele-vision*. London: BFI, 1996.

Wittich, Walter Arno, and John Guy Fowlkes. *Audio-Visual Paths to Learning*. New York: Harper, 1946.

Wolf, Eric. *Europe and the People Without History*. Berkeley: University of California Press, 1982.

Wood, Denis. *The Power of Maps*. New York: Guilford, 1992.

Wood, Richard, ed. *Film and Propaganda in America: A Documentary History. Volume I: World War I*. New York: Greenwood, 1990.

World Health Organization. *Introducing WHO*. Geneva: WHO, 1976.

Wylie, Philip. *Generation of Vipers*. New York: Rinehart, 1955.

Yoshimoto, Mitsuhiro. "Real Virtuality." In *Global/Local: Cultural Production and the Transnational Imaginary*. Ed. by Rob Wilson and Wimal Dissana-yake. Durham: Duke University Press, 1996.

Zinsser, Hans. *Rats, Lice and History: A Study in Biography*. Boston: Little, Brown, 1934.

Filmography

About AIDS. Prod. by Health Education Video Unit, Leistershire Health Authority. 1986.

AIDS. Prod. by Health Education Technologies. 1987.

AIDS and Health-Care Workers: A Video Report. Prod. by U.S. Department of Health and Human Services. 1988.

AIDS and Other Epidemics. Prod. by Films for the Humanities. 1990.

The AIDS Antibody Test. Prod. by Adair and Armstrong and San Francisco AIDS Foundation. 1987.

AIDS: Changing the Rules. Prod. by AIDS FILMS, Inc. and WETA-TV, Washington, D.C. 1987.

AIDS: Everything You and Your Family Need to Know . . . But Were Afraid to Ask. Dir. by Vincent Stafford. Prod. by HBO. 1988.

AIDS Hits Home. Prod. by Dan Rather/CBS. 1986.

AIDS: On the Front Line. Prod. by Olivier Video. 1987.

The AIDS Quarterly. Prod. by Peter Jennings/ABC/WGBH. Spring 1990.

AIDS: The Surgeon General's Update. Prod. by Consultants International and U.S. Office of the Assistant Secretary for Health and Surgeon General. 1987.

AIDS . . . What YOU Need to Know: The Surgeon General's Report to the Nation. Prod. by Consultants International. 1987.

Alien Nation. Prod. by 20th Century Fox. 1989–90.

And the Band Played On. Dir. by Roger Spottiswoode. Prod. by HBO. 1993.

The Andromeda Strain. Dir. by Robert Wise. Prod. by Universal. 1971.

The Architecture of Doom. Dir. by Peter Cohen. Prod. by Svenska Filminstitutet. 1989.

Are You Fit to Marry? Dir. by W. H. Stafford. Prod. by Quality Amusement Corp. 1927.

Asian Influenza Vaccination. Prod. by U.S. Public Health Service/Communicable Disease Center. 1957.

BaadAssss Cinema: A Bold Look at 70's Blaxploitation Films. Dir. by Isaac Julien. Prod. by IFC Films/Docurama. 2002.

Biohazard Outbreak. Videogame. Prod. by Eiichiro Sasaki, Capcom. 2004.

Birth of a Baby. Dir. by A. E. Christie. Prod. by James Skirball. 1937.

Blow Out. Dir. by Brian De Palma. Prod. by Cinema 77/Filmways. 1981.

The Business of Health. Prod. by U.S. Information Agency. NARA: 306.6608. n.d.

Can AIDS Be Stopped? Prod. by WGBH. 1986.

Capitol Story. Prod. by U.S. Public Health Service. NARA: 59.23. 1945.

The Case History of Lucy X: A Story Based on an Actual Case History Taken from the Files of the Association. Prod. by National Tuberculosis Association. 1945.

Choose to Live. Prod. by U.S. Public Health Service/American Society for Control of Cancer/U.S. Department of Agriculture Extension Service. NARA: 90.1. 1940.

Chorea. Prod. by Neurological Cinematographic Atlas. Ed. Adolf Nichtenhauser. 1944.

Cloud in the Sky. Prod. by National Tuberculosis Association. NARA: NTA-NTA-2. 1939.

The Coming Plague. Prod. by Turner Original Productions. 1997.

Communicating for Health. Prod. by U.S. Public Health Service. 1985.

The Conversation. Dir. by Francis Ford Coppola. Prod. by American Zoetrope/Paramount. 1974.

The Crazies. Dir. by George Romero. Prod. by Pittsburgh/Cambist Films. 1973.

Criminal at Large. Prod. by Office of Malaria Control in War Areas. NARA: 90.28. 1945.

Damaged Goods. Dir. by Phil Stone. Prod. by Criterion Pictures. 1937.

Damaged Lives. Dir. by Edgar Ulmer. Prod. by Weldon Co. 1933.

Dance, Little Children. Prod. by Centron/U.S. Public Health Service. 1965.

Dark Skies. Prod. by Columbia Pictures Television. 1996–97.

Dawn of the Dead. Dir. by Zack Snyder. Prod. by Strike/New Amsterdam. 2004.

The Day the Earth Stood Still. Dir. by Robert Wise. Prod. by 20th Century Fox. 1951.

Destination Moon. Dir. by Irving Pichel. Prod. by George Pal. 1950.

Disaster Aid: Public Health Aspects. Prod. by U.S. Department of Health, Education and Welfare/U.S. Public Health Service/Centers for Disease Control. NARA: 286.44. 1955.

A Doctor for Ardaknos. Prod. by International Communication Agency/U.S. Information Agency. NARA: 306.50. n.d. [c. 1948–1959].

The End of the Road. Prod. by American Social Hygiene Association. NARA: ASHA-ASHA-200; NARA: 200.200. 1919.

Enemy X. Prod. by U.S. Public Health Service/American Society for Control of Cancer/CBS. NARA: 90.3. 1942.

An Epidemic of Fear: AIDS in the Workplace. Prod. by San Francisco AIDS Foundation and Pacific Bell. 1987.

An Epidemic of Histoplasmosis Associated with an Urban Starling Roost. Prod. by Kansas University Medical Center/Communicable Disease Center. 1961.

The Epidemiology of Murine Typhus. Prod. by U.S. Public Health Service/Communicable Disease Center. 1948.

The Eternal Fight. Prod. by United Nations Film Board/Madeline Carroll Films. 1948.

Evil Wind Out. Dir. by James Blue. Prod. by U.S. Information Agency. NARA: 306.338. 1963.

The Fight Against the Communicable Diseases. Prod. by U.S. Public Health Service. NARA: 90.30. 1950.

The Fight for Life. Dir. by Pare Lorentz. Prod. by U.S. Film Service. 1940.

Fight Syphilis. Dir. by Owen Murray. Prod. by U.S. Public Health Service. NARA: 90.5; NARA: III-M-942. 1941.

Filariasis in British Guiana. Prod. by British Guiana-U.S.A. Technical Assistance Development Organization/U.S. Agency for International Development. 1963.

First Aid Treatment after Exposure to Syphilis. Prod. by Bray Studios/U.S. Public Health Service. NARA: 90.27. 1924.

The Fly as a Disease Carrier. Prod. by Bray Studios/U.S. Public Health Service. NARA: 90.23. 1924.

Food Sanitation: Food Poisoning on Shipboard. Prod. by U.S. Navy Training Film/Caravel Films. 1951.

For Health and Happiness. Prod. by U.S. Information Agency. NARA: 306.2712. n.d. [c. 1920s].

For the Nation's Health. Prod. by Communicable Disease Center. 1952.

General Personal Hygiene. Prod. by Bray Studios/U.S. Public Health Service. NARA: 90.26. 1924.

Giant in the Sun. Prod. by Northern Nigeria Information Service. NARA: 286.105. 1957.

Growing Up in the Age of AIDS. Prod. by Peter Jennings/ABC News. 1992.

Guess Who's Coming to Dinner? Dir. by Stanley Kramer. Prod. by Columbia. 1967.

Guilty Parents. Dir. by John Townley. Prod. by Jay Dee Kay. 1934.

Hackers. Dir. by Iain Softley. Prod. by United Artists. 1995.

Hand Ditching for Malaria Control. Prod. by U.S. Public Health Service/Centers for Disease Control. 1949.

A Handful of Soil. Prod. by U.S. Information Service. NARA: 306.4055. n.d.

Handwashing in Patient Care. Prod. by U.S. Public Health Service. 1961.

Health for Youth. Prod. by National Youth Administration/U.S. Public Health Service. NARA: 119.17. 1941.

The Health Fraud Racket. Prod. by Federal Drug Administration/U.S. Department of Health, Education and Welfare/Audio Productions. 1966.

Health in Our Community. Prod. by Encyclopedia Britannica. 1959.

Health Is a Victory. Prod. by American Social Hygiene Association. NARA: ASHA-ASHA-198; NARA: 200.198. 1942.

Hemolytic Streptococcus Control. Prod. by Wilding Picture Productions/U.S. Navy. 1945.

High School Girl. Dir. by Crane Wilbur. Prod. by Foy Productions. 1934.

Hospital Sepsis: A Communicable Disease. Prod. by Churchill-Wexler Films. 1959.

How Disease Is Spread. Prod. by Bray Studios/u.s. Public Health Service. NARA: 90.20. 1924.

How Plants and Animals Cause Disease. Prod. by Bray Studios/u.s. Public Health Service. NARA: 90.18. 1924.

How the Mosquito Spreads Disease. Prod. by Bray Studios/u.s. Public Health Service. NARA: 90.22. 1924.

How to Prevent Diseases. Prod. by Bray Studios/u.s. Public Health Service. NARA: 90.21. 1924.

Human Wreckage: They Must Be Told. Prod. by Cinema Service Corp. 1938.

I Dress the Wound. Prod. by Churchill-Wexler. 1960.

I Married a Monster from Outer Space. Dir. by Gene Fowler Jr. Prod. by Paramount. 1958.

In Defense of the Nation. Prod. by Jam Handy/u.s. Public Health Service. NARA: 90.6. 1941.

The Innocent Party. Prod. by Centron. 1959.

Interdependence of Living Things. Prod. by u.s. Public Health Service. NARA: 90.4. 1924.

The Invaders. Prod. by Quinn Martin. 1967–68.

Invaders from Mars. Dir. by William Cameron Menzies. Prod. by National Pictures. 1953.

Invasion of the Body Snatchers. Dir. by Donald Siegel. Prod. by Allied Artists/Walter Wanger. 1956.

Invisible Invaders. Dir. by Edward L. Cahn. Prod. by Premium Pictures. 1959.

Isolation Technique. Prod. by u.s. Navy. 1944.

It Came from Outer Space. Dir. by Jack Arnold. Prod. by Universal. 1953.

It Conquered the World. Dir. by Roger Corman. Prod. by American International Pictures/Sunset. 1956.

The Jazz Singer. Dir. by Alan Crosland. Prod. by Warner Bros. 1927.

Les Joyeux Microbes. Dir. by Emile Cohl. Prod. by Gaumont, France. 1909.

Karate Kids. Prod. by National Film Board of Canada/World Health Organization/UNICEF/Pan-American Health Organization. 1990.

Keep Clean, Stay Well. Prod. by Agency for International Development. NARA: 286.213. 1964.

Keep 'em Out. Prod. by Stark/U.S. Public Health Service. 1942.

Know for Sure. Dir. by Lewis Milestone. Prod. by Research Council of the Academy of Motion Picture Arts and Sciences/U.S. Public Health Service. NARA: 90.7. 1941.

Laboratory Control in Milk Sanitation. Prod. by U.S. Public Health Service/ Communicable Disease Center. 1951.

Laboratory Design for Microbiological Safety. Prod. by U.S. Public Health Service. 1966.

Let My People Live. Prod. by National Tuberculosis Association. NARA: NTA-NTA-232; NARA: 200.232. 1944.

. . . Like Any Other Patient. Prod. by Regional Learning Resources Services, St. Louis/VAMC. 1989.

Local Health Problems in War Industry Areas. Prod. by Division of Public Education, New York State Department of Health. 1942.

Magic Bullets. Prod. by U.S. Public Health Service/Warner Brothers. NARA: 90.8. 1940.

Malaria. Prod. by U.S. Public Health Service. NARA: 90.29. 1944.

Malaria Eradication. Prod. by U.S. Information Agency. NARA: 306.5547. 1958.

Man Learns to Heal. Prod. by U.S. Information Agency. NARA: 306.5536. 1957.

Medical Service in the Invasion of Normandy. Prod. by U.S. War Department/ Army Pictorial Service. 1944.

Merchant Marine Rest Centers. Prod. by Maritime Commission. NARA: 178.41. 1944.

Middletown Goes to War. Prod. by National Tuberculosis Association. NARA: NTA-NTA-8; NARA: 200.8. 1942.

Military Sanitation: Disposal of Human Waste. Official Training Film. Prod. by War Department/U.S. Army Signal Corps. 1943.

Mimic. Dir. by Guillermo del Toro. Prod. by Dimension/Miramax. 1997.

Miracle in Tonga. Prod. by U.S. Public Health Service/Centers for Disease Control. 1965.

Miracle of Birth. 1930s.

Mission: Impossible II. Dir. by John Woo. Prod. by Paramount. 2000.

The Mississippi Valley Disease: Histoplasmosis. Prod. by University of Kansas/ Centers for Disease Control. 1956.

Modern Motherhood. Dir. by Dwain Esper. Prod. by Roadshow Attractions Co. 1934.

Mom and Dad. Dir. by Kroger Babb. Prod. by Hygienic Productions. 1944.

A Monthly Review from Europe. Mutual Security Agency Newsreel, vol. 1, no. 3. Prod. by World Health Organization. NARA: 306.103C. 1952.

The Mosquito. Combat Film Report, no. 157. Prod. by Army Air Forces. NARA: 18-C-157. 1945.

The Naked Truth. Dir. by Fred Sullivan. Prod. by Samuel Cummins/Public Welfare Pictures Co. American Social Hygiene Assoc. 1927.

Nanook of the North. Dir. by Robert J. Flaherty. Prod. by Robert J. Flaherty. 1922.

The National Library of Medicine. Prod. by U.S. Public Health Service. 1963.

The New Frontier. Prod. by USDA/Federal Emergency Relief Administration. 1934.

On the Firing Line: A Travel-Tour to Scenes of the Fight Against Tuberculosis. Prod. by National Tuberculosis Association/Courier Productions. NARA: NTA-NTA-I. 1939.

Other Faces of AIDS. Prod. by Maryland Public Television. 1989.

Our Immune System. Prod. by National Geographic Society. 1988.

Outbreak. Dir. by Wolfgang Petersen. Prod. by Warner Brothers. 1995.

An Outbreak of Salmonella Infection. Prod. by U.S. Public Health Service/Communicable Disease Center. 1954.

Pandora's Clock. Prod. by NBC Telefilm. 1996.

Panic in the Streets. Dir. by Elia Kazan. Prod. by 20th Century Fox. 1950.

The Parallax View. Dir. by Alan Pakula. Prod. by Paramount. 1974.

Passport to Health. Prod. by U.S. Information Agency. NARA: 306.6851. n.d. [c. 1950].

Pepperbird Land. Prod. by Griff Davis. NARA: 286.298. 1958.

Personal Hygiene for Girls. Prod. by Bray Studios/U.S. Public Health Service. NARA: 90.24. 1924.

Personal Hygiene for Women. Prod. by U.S. Navy/Audio Productions. 1943.

Personal Hygiene for Young Men. Prod. by Bray Studios/U.S. Public Health Service. NARA: 90.25. 1924.

Pitfalls of Passion. Dir. by Leonard Livingstone. Prod. by S. S. Millard. 1927.

The Plow That Broke the Plains. Dir. by Pare Lorentz. Prod. by u.s. Film Service. 1936.

Power and the Land. Prod. by USDA Rural Electrification Administration. 1940.

The President's Analyst. Dir. by Theodore J. Flicker. Prod. by Panpiper/Paramount. 1967.

Prevention of the Introduction of Diseases from Abroad. Prod. by u.s. Public Health Service/Bray Studios. 1946.

Public Health. Prod. by u.s. Information Agency. NARA: 306.6036. n.d. [c. 1950].

Public Health: A Case of the Blues. Prod. by u.s. Information Agency/Owen Murphy. NARA: 306.6016. n.d. [ca. 1950].

Public Health in New York State. Prod. by Division of Public Health Education, New York State Department of Health. 1937.

Public Health: WHO Conference in Congo. Prod. by u.s. Information Agency. NARA: 306.6037. n.d.

The Rat Problem. Prod. by u.s. Army/u.s. Public Health Service/Communicable Disease Center. 1950.

Les Rayons Roentgen (aka *A Novice at X-Rays*). Dir. by Georges Méliès. 1897.

Red Dawn. Dir. by John Milius. Prod. by Sidney Beckerman/United Artists. 1984.

Reefer Madness. Dir. by Louis Gasnier. Prod. by G&H. 1938.

The Reproductive System. Prod. by Jacob Sarnoff. 1924–27?

Reward Unlimited. Prod. by u.s. Public Health Service/Office of War Information/War Activities Committee. NARA: 90.0. 1944.

The Rhesus Monkeys of Santiago Island, Puerto Rico. Prod. by u.s. Public Health Service. 1963.

The River. Dir. by Pare Lorentz. Prod. by u.s. Film Service. 1938.

Rocketship X-M. Dir. by Kurt Neumann. Prod. by Lippert Pictures. 1950.

Roswell. Prod. by 20th Century Fox/WB. 1999–2002.

Routine Admission Chest X-Ray in General Hospitals. Prod. by u.s. Public Health Service. 1946.

Runaway Virus. Dir. by Jeff Bleckner. 2000.

Rural Nurse: A Pilot Project in El Salvador. Prod. by Agency for International Development. NARA: 286.133. 1954.

Rx: Innovation. Prod. by U.S. Public Health Service/U.S. Department of Health, Education, and Welfare. 1966.

Safe. Dir. by Todd Haynes. Prod. by American Playhouse/Channel Four/ Good Machine. 1995.

Sanitary Devices in the Field, Part I: Safe Water, Clean Bodies, Clothes and Mess Gear. Prod. by U.S. Army. 1950.

Sanitary Devices in the Field, Part II: Disposal of Wastes. Prod. by U.S. Army. 1950.

Sanitation Techniques in Rat Control. Prod. by U.S. Army/U.S. Public Health Service/Communicable Disease Center. 1950.

Save a Day! Prod. by Federal Security Agency/U.S. Public Health Service. NARA: 90.11. 1941.

The Science of Life. Motion Picture Series. Prod. by Bray Studios/U.S. Public Health Service. NARA: 90.18–27. 1924.

Sex and the Scientist. Prod. by Indiana University Audio-Visual Center. 1989.

Sex Hygiene. Prod. by Audio Productions [for U.S. Navy]. 1942.

Shaft. Dir. by Gordon Parks. Prod. by MGM. 1971.

Shipboard Inspection by Medical Department Personnel: Food Storage. Prod. by U.S. Navy/Producers Film Studios. 1958.

The Silent Invader. Prod. by Westinghouse Broadcasting/U.S. Public Health Service. 1957.

Sins of the Fathers. Prod. by Canada Motion Picture Council. 1948.

The Stand. Prod. by ABC. 1994.

The Story of My Life, By Tee Bee. Prod. by National Tuberculosis Association. NARA: NTA-NTA-5; NARA: 200.6. 1932.

Striking Back Against Rabies. Prod. by Federal Security Agency/U.S. Public Health Service/Communicable Disease Center. 1950.

Sweet Sweetback's Baadasssss Song. Dir. by Melvin Van Peebles. Prod. by Yeah. 1971.

Talkin' About AIDS. Prod. by Canadian Broadcasting Company/Atlantic Films. 1990.

Them! Dir. by Gordon Douglas. Prod. by Warner Brothers. 1954.

They Do Come Back. Dir. by Edward G. Ulmer. Prod. by National Tuberculosis Association. NARA: NTA-NTA-7; NARA: 200.7. 1940.

Three Counties Against Syphilis. Prod. by U.S. Public Health Service/Department of Agriculture. NARA: 90.12. 1938.

Three Days of the Condor. Dir. by Sydney Pollack. Prod. by Dino de Laurentiis/Paramount. 1975.

Thumbs Up for Kids! AIDS Education. Prod. by KTVU-TV, Media Express, Inc., AIMS Media. 1989.

To the People of the United States. Dir. by Arthur Lubin. Prod. by Walter Wanger/U.S. Public Health Service. NARA: 90.13. 1944.

Tomorrow's Epidemic. Prod. by World Health Organization/Actua Film Geneva. 1980.

Tropical Disease Investigation in Africa. Prod. by U.S. Public Health Service. 1957.

Tsutsugamushi: Prevention. Prod. by U.S. Navy/Audio Productions. 1945.

Twelve Monkeys. Dir. by Terry Gilliam. Prod. by Universal. 1995.

28 Days Later . . . Dir. by Danny Boyle. Prod. by British Film Council, Canal +, DNA Films, and Figment Films. 2002.

The Venereal Diseases. Prod. by American Social Hygiene Assoc. 1928.

A Venezuelan Equine Encephalitis Epidemic in Columbia. Prod. by U.S. Public Health Service. 1968.

Virus. Dir. by John Bruno. Prod. by BBC/Dark Horse. 1999.

Le voyage dans la lune (aka *A Trip to the Moon*). Dir. by Georges Méliès. 1898.

The War of the Worlds. Dir. by Byron Haskin. Prod. by Paramount. 1953.

What Price Innocence? Dir. by Willard Mack. Prod. by Columbia. 1933.

What the Doctor Ordered. Prod. by John Burch/BBC TV/Churchill Films. 1986.

What You Should Know About AIDS. Prod. by Centers for Disease Control. 1987.

The Wizard of Oz. Dir. by Victor Fleming. Prod. by MGM. 1939.

The Work of the Public Health Service. Prod. by U.S. Public Health Service/Bray Studios. 1936.

The X Files. Exec. Prod., Chris Carter. Prod. by 20th Century Fox Television. 1993–2002.

You Can Be Safe From X-Rays. Prod. by Federal Security Agency/U.S. Public Health Service/Communicable Disease Center. 1952.

Your Health Department. Prod. by National Motion Pictures Co. 1941.

Index

Page numbers in italics indicate illustrations.

48–50, 59, 66–76, 118–19, 207n4, 207n9; animation, 208n14; anthropomorphized disease, 122, 181–82, 187; autonomous bacteria in a hospital ventilation system and, 149–54; in documentary-style footage, 85–86; epidemiological mapping, 129–31; integration of, with indexical representations, 156–57, 175–76, 185–88, 190–91, 194–95; special effects, 90, 191; using digitized technology, 157, 167. *See also* cinematic techniques; digital technology; indexical visualizations of disease

Asian influenza, 219n45

aural representations of disease, 10, 21, 49–50, 60, 64, 67, 74–78

bacteriology, 26, 50–53, 211n4, 215n4

Baudrillard, Jean, 130, 133–34, 217n29, 219–20n8

Bazin, André, 49, 206–7n3, 207n6

Beau Geste, 34

Bennell, Dr. Miles (character), 91–97

Bin Laden, Osama, 80

Biography of a Germ, 176

Biohazard Outbreak (videogame), 176

Black, Gregory, 42

Black, Jeremy, 217n27

Black Stork, The, 41, 206n63, 207n8

blaxploitation movement, 169–70, 174, 220nn19, 21

Blow Out, 219n7

Borges, Jorge Luis, 130

Bray Studios, 4, 57, 208n19, 210n39

Brokaw, Tom, 178

Can AIDS Be Stopped?, 221n29

cartography. *See* mapping

Cartwright, Lisa, 54

categories of difference. *See* class; gender norms; racial factors

Catholic Legion of Decency, 34, 40–41, 201n18, 206n61

censorship, 24–31; First Amendment protection of film and, 202n26; Progressive reform movement and, 26–27; under ratings system of 1968, 18–19, 168–69; self-regulation by the film industry and, 31, 41, 203n34, 204n37, 205n40; of U.S. government propaganda films, 24. *See also* Production Code

Centers for Disease Control and Prevention (CDC), 2, 124–25; audiovisual production activities of, 126–28, 216n20; Epidemiological Intelligence Service (EIS) of, 125–26; *The Fight Against the Communicable Diseases* and, 139–40, 140

Charters, Werrett Wallace, 203n34

Chase, Canon William Sheafe, 202n32

children. *See* spectatorship

cinematic techniques, 11, 13–17; animated maps, 8–9, 64–65, 73–75, 102; animation, 49–50, 62, 63, 64, 67, 72, 207n9, 208n14; close-ups, 6–7, 21, 21–22; digital imaging, 17; documentary stock footage, 84–86, 88–90, 118–20, 149, 211n10; enlarged microscopic cinematography, 53, 54–55; enlargements, 54; fast and slow motion, 54; film within a film technique, 85, 211–12n12; microscopic animation, 208n19; newsreel-style montage, 86, 88; point-of-view camerawork, 99–101, 100, 185–87, 213n31; reductions of the image, 54; 16 mm film, 13; soundtracks, 103; special effects, 85–86, 90, 105–6, 118–20,

cinematic techniques (*continued*)
191, 211n11; split-screen composition,
157; synchronized sound, 27–30, 42–
43, 201n18; theremin soundtracks,
101; three-dimensional film, 213n31;
unity of image and sound, 77–78,
210nn44–46; video technology, 13,
168, 171–72; voiceover, 10, 21, 49–50,
60, 64, 67, 72, 76–78, 88, 207n9. *See
also* mapping; visual representations
of disease

civil rights, 12

Civil War, 81

class, 3, 7–9; in alien invasion films,
92–93, 212n20; assimilation of
immigrants and, 26–27, 205n52;
domestic sphere of middle classes
and, 7–8; immigrant contagions
and, 19–24, 37–38, 199n3, 199–
200n5; impact of, on film viewing,
32–33, 204n36; middle-class whiteness as normative, 8, 53, 78, 92–93,
212n20; public sphere of the working
class and, 7–9; of representations of
disease, 8

Coming Plague, The (Garrett), 177,
221n29, 223n54

Communicable Disease Center, 124–25.
See also Centers for Disease Control
and Prevention (CDC)

Communism, 12; anti-Communist
films and, 215n52; disease metaphors
and, 94–95, 211n7; influence of mass
culture and, 96; physical fitness and,
81; rhetoric of invasion by invisible
enemies and, 16–17, 82–83, 116,
212n21, 217–18n30; science fiction
allegories of, 16, 94–95, 119, 215n52

computer virus rhetoric, 14, 80–81,
192–96

conspiracy narratives, 16–17, 122, 131–
54, 212n21, 217–18n30; abstracted
representations of disease and, 148–
54, 168, 174–76; dialectic of visibility
and invisibility and, 131–32, 138–39,
167, 218nn32–33; documentary format of *The Andromeda Strain* and,
156–60, 167, 219n4; injection panic
and, 218n34; linkage of national
penetration with homosexual panic
and, 157, 163–66, 177–88, 219–20n8;
literary examples of, 217–18n30; paranoia and, 137–38; reconfiguration of
gender norms and, 156; search for
bodily integrity and, 160, 219n7; self-
surveillance and, 143–44; transnational transportation and disinfection
and, 58, 137–39, 143–44; universality
of infection and, 149, 154

Conversation, The, 219n7

Cook, Robin, 177

Corning Incorporated's Hazelton Research Products, 179–80

Crazies, The, 135, 210n43, 218n34

Creel Committee, 209nn30–31

"Crisis in the Hot Zone" (Preston),
179–80

Cumming, Hugh S., 58

Dark Skies (TV series), 176

Dawn of the Dead, 176

Day the Earth Stood Still, The, 101, 119

Destination Moon, 84–86, 211nn9, 11

Devil's Flu, The (Davies), 176

digital technology, 155–91; anthropomorphized virus and, 181–82, 187;
competing versions of truth and,
160–61; computer viruses and, 14,
80–81, 192–96; documentary format
and, 156–60, 167, 219n4; elimination

of gap between fiction and reality and, 178–79, 194–95; elimination of gap between visible and invisible and, 167, 193–94; fetishizing in *The Andromeda Strain* and, 157–58, 166–67; integration of indexical and artificial representations and, 167, 194–95; invisibility of racial and sexual identity and, 193–94, 224n7; national penetration by viruses and, 193–94; in *Outbreak*, 175–76, 181–82, 185–88; predictive mapping and, 189, 223n53; realism of, 156–58

diseases: bubonic plague, 21–22, 58, 123, 199n3; cholera, 58, 72, 73–74, 123; Ebola virus, 155, 177–88, 222n41; foot-and-mouth disease, 1, 14; influenza, 139–40, 144–48, 219n45; malaria, 58; pneumonic plague, 20–21, 58; polio, 111, 214n45, 216n20; severe acute respiratory syndrome (SARS), 1, 14, 197n1, 222n46; smallpox, 72; typhus fever, 66–76, 140–44, 199–200n5; venereal, 56–57, 135–38, 208n25, 210n39, 215–16n7; yellow fever, 54, 58, 72, 123, 138. *See also* AIDS education; *Hemolytic Streptococcus Control*

Doane, Mary Ann, 77, 210n44, 218n38

documentary film, definition, 43–44. *See also* educational films

Doherty, Thomas, 28–29

Duffy, John, 25–26, 201n20, 211n4

Ebola virus, 155, 177–88, 222n41

economic factors: gendered consumer culture and, 9–10; production of public health films and, 25–26

educational films: from the Centers for Disease Control and Prevention (CDC), 125–28, 216n20; cinematic authority and, 207n5; "compensating moral value" requirement of, 42, 45; definition of, 43–44; early public health films, 55; economic limitations of, 25–26; impact of movie content of, 37–38; impact of the Production Code on, 20, 24–31, 40–46, 200n7; mixed-gender audiences of, 40–41; narrative structure of, 19; nontheatrical film definition of, 41–43; on polio, 111, 214n45, 216n20; produced by U.S. government, 24; prohibited from theaters, 18–19, 41–43, 199n1; promotion of patriotism of, 209nn30–31; propaganda films and, 24; realism of, 24–25, 30–31, 33–34, 84; replacement of, by television and video, 168, 172–75; "Safety First" campaign of, 55; search for imagery of contagion of, 79–80; Spanish American War footage and, 53–54; stylistic overlap of, with alien invasion films, 83–91; theory of backlash and, 169–70; world health training films and, 126–28. *See also* AIDS education; public health departments

Encyclopedia Britannica, 200n7

entertainment films: "compensating moral value" component of, 42, 45; impact of sound on, 27, 30, 77–78, 201n18, 210nn44–46; moral contagion and, 18, 24–31, 35–36, 134–35, 195; pre-Code styles of, 27–29, 50, 207n8; realism of, 19, 84–91, 105–6, 212nn18–19. *See also* alien invasion films; conspiracy narratives

Epidemic of Fear, An, 223n54

Epidemiological Intelligence Service (EIS), 125–26

Grierson, John, 43–44

Growing Up in the Age of AIDS, 223n54

Guerrero, Ed, 169, 220n21

Guess Who's Coming to Dinner?, 169, 220n16

Gunning, Tom, 54

Guns, Germs, and Steel: The Fates of Human Societies (Diamond), 176–77

Hackers, 176

Hall (protagonist of *The Andromeda Strain*), 161–66, 219n6

Hart, Kylo-Patrick R., 175

Hays, Will, 35–36, 203–4n35

Hays Office. *See* Motion Picture Producers and Distributors of America

Hazelton Research Products, 179–80

health education, 25–26

Health Organization of the League of Nations, 124

Hemolytic Streptococcus Control, 15, 48, 59–66, 62–63, 76, 135; animated arrows in, 62, 63, 64; animated maps in, 73–74; fears of homosexuality in, 64, 106, 215–16n7; gap between image and sound in, 60, 209n36; homosocial environment in, 61–64, 180; microscopic animation in, 208n19; voiceover narrative in, 60, 64, 209n36

historic contexts, 12, 50–59; of early educational films, 55; invention of cinema and, 50–51, 54; of public health, 50–51, 81–83; of world health, 123–28, 215n2, 216n17

HIV (human immunodeficiency virus). *See* AIDS education

Hollywood Production Code. *See* Production Code

homosexuality: AIDS activist videos and, 170; body doubling in alien invasion films and, 104–11, 114–15; conflated with threat of contamination, 156–57; epistemology of the closet and, 105–9, 114–15; fears of homosexual contagion and, 17, 64, 96–97, 103–4, 119, 132–33, 214n38; homoerotic spectacle and, 157, 161–66; homophobia and, 155–58; homosocial environments and, 61–64, 180, 215–16n7; invisibility and, 109–18; penetration panic and, 49, 104, 119, 132–33, 157, 160–66, 177–88, 218n34, 219–20n8. *See also* AIDS education

Hoover, J. Edgar, 95

Hospital Sepsis, 148–54, 150–53, 176, 208n19

Hot Zone, The (Preston), 177–82

How Disease is Spread, 4–10, 5, 9, 57, 65, 198n10, 210n39; animated maps in, 73–74, 135; cinematic techniques of, 6–9; class factors of, 6–10; definition of disease carriers in, 7–8; eugenics movement and, 5–6; gender norms in, 6–8, 10

human body, 16; anxious juncture of modernization and disease and, 47–48; doubling of, in alien invasion films, 104–11, 114–15, 214n37; fears of homosexual contagion and, 17, 64, 96–97, 103–4, 119, 132–33, 214n38; homoerotic spectacle in *The Andromeda Strain* and, 157, 161–66; indexical visualizations of disease and, 3, 44–45, 47–50, 197n2, 206–7n3; marks of possession by aliens on, 104, 110, 214n44; metaphors of geopolitical invasion and, 114–22, 132–34, 163–66, 175–79; objectification of the female body and, 156; possession of, in alien invasion films, 102–11, 121–22, 132–34, 212n19;

human body (*continued*)
status of boundaries of, 65–66; use of close-up techniques on, 6–7. *See also* sexuality
human immunodeficiency virus. *See* AIDS education

Illness as Metaphor (Sontag), 211n7
images of contagion. *See* visual representations of disease
"Imagination of Disaster, The" (Sontag), 86–87
I Married a Monster from Outer Space, 101, 104, 109, 111–19, 113, 214n37
immigration: assimilation and, 26–27, 205n52; entry inspections and, 51, 98, 124; ethnic contagions and, 19–24, 37–38, 52–53, 98, 199n3, 199–200n5, 208n13, 215n7; fears of terrorism and, 80; following World War One, 56; Immigration Act of 1924 and, 56; origins of public health and, 51; quarantines and, 10, 124
indexical visualizations of disease, 3, 44–50, 118–19, 197n2, 206–7n3, 207nn4, 9; in documentary-style footage, 85–86; integration of, with artificial representations, 156–57, 175–76, 185–88, 190–91, 194–95; link between contagion and identity and, 66; mapping and, 123, 128–35, 152–54, 216–17n26, 217n27, 218nn32–33; racial contagion and, 66–76; sexualized transmission of disease and, 59–66, 76; using digital technology and, 157, 167. *See also* artificial representations of disease; race; sexuality
international health organizations. *See* world health
Invaders from Mars, 101, 103, 104, 109–10, 119

Invaders, The (television series), 213n30
Invasion of the Body Snatchers, 16, 91–97, 93, 101, 116, 119; as allegory of communism, 94–95; body doubling in, 104–11, 214n37; Communist conspiracy theories and, 212n19; dependence on normative social structures and, 92–93, 212n20; documentary stock footage and, 211n10; gap between image and sound and, 60, 91–94, 209–10n37, 212n19; unreliable narrator of, 91–92
Invisible Enemy, The: A Natural History of Viruses, 176
Invisible Invaders, 90, 119, 121
It Came from Outer Space, 98–101, 100, 104, 119, 213n31
It Conquered the World, 101–4, 107–8, 119, 214n37

Jazz Singer, The, 27
Johnson, Lyndon B., 127–28
Joyeux Microbes, Les, 208n14

Kennedy, John F., 217–18n30
King, Geoff, 125, 130, 132, 217n29
Kinsella, James, 170
Kinsey, Alfred C., reports, 96
Kleinschmidt, H. E., 200n6
Knee, Adam, 85–86, 115–18
Know for Sure, 208n19
Koop, C. Everett, 223n50
Korean War, 126
Kramer, Larry, 221n24
Kraut, Alan, 52

Lacan, Jacques, 160, 219n7
League of Nations, 124
. . . *Like Any Other Patient*, 171, 172–73
Lindbergh, Charles, 57

camerawork in, 185–87; representation of homosexuality in, 184–85, 222n48; species jumping in, 182–85, 223n52

Palomar Observatory telescope, 103, 213n34

Pandora's Clock, 176

Panic in the Streets, 19–24, 23, 45, 199n2; ethnic markers in, 20–21; injection panic in, 132–33, 218n34; narrative tension in, 20–21

Paramount decrees of 1948, 168

Patton, Cindy, 185–86

Payne Fund Studies, 31–40, 203n34, 205n40; critiques of, 203–4n35; discourse of contagion and, 37–39; funding of, 202n32; linkage of education and realism in, 33–34; moral impact of spectatorship in, 32–39; movies as "school of conduct" and, 36–37; *Movies, Delinquency, and Crime* (Forman) and, 36–37; *Our Movie Made Children* (Forman) and, 32–39

Peirce, C. S., 206–7n3

penicillin, 81–82, 211n4

Pernick, Martin, 41–42, 55, 207n8

Personal Hygiene for Girls, 4

Peters, C. J., 179–80

Plague Time, 176

postmodernity: conspiracy narratives and, 131–54, 217–18n30, 218nn32–33; gendered anxiety about mass culture and, 134, 219–20n8; mapping and, 130–31, 217nn27–29, 218n33

post–World War Two period: antibiotics in, 81–82, 167, 211n4; anti-Communist films in, 215n52; blurred boundaries between reality and image in, 133–34; cross-pollination of genres in, 45–46; gender struggles in, 214–15n46; global surveillance project in, 51, 73–75, 95, 122–28, 142–44, 157, 218–19n43; mobile privatization in, 95–96; paranoid fiction in, 133; public school use of audiovisual technology in, 26, 45, 201n10; reconfiguration of gender norms in, 156; use of term "documentaries" in, 43. *See also* Communism; world health

post–World War Two public health films, 2, 11–17, 58–59; abstracted representations of disease in, 148–54, 168, 174–76; animation in, 66–76; anthropomorphized disease in, 122; artificial representations of disease in, 48–50, 59; cinematic authority in, 207n5; conspiracy narrative form in, 122–23, 131–54, 217–18n30, 218nn32–33; cross-pollination of genres of, 45–46; dialectic of visibility and invisibility in, 14–17, 97–104, 112–21, 128–35, 138, 149, 167, 212n19; fears of homosexual contagion in, 17, 64, 96–97, 103–11, 119, 214n38; globalized context of, 10–12, 65–66, 90, 135, 158, 198n15; homosocial environments in, 61–64; indexical visualizations of disease in, 3, 47–50, 59–66, 197n2, 206–7n3; injection panic in, 132–33, 218n34, 219–20n8; military training films and, 33, 57, 135–38, 208n25, 210n39; racial and ethnic otherness in, 10, 11–12, 16, 197–98n9, 215nn4, 6–7; realism of, 84, 105–6; replacement of, by television and video, 172–75; sexual norms in, 10, 11–12, 16; Third World origins of disease in, 128–29, 136,

and, 22, 57–59, 67–72, 210n42; use
of pesticides and, 58; "visualization
equals inoculation" formula and,
179; white western males as normative and, 78. *See also* AIDS education;
mapping; visual representations of
disease

World Health Organization (WHO),
2, 75; creation of, 124; health surveillance networks and, 157; as icon
in science fiction films, 86–88; *A
Monthly Review from Europe* and, 140–
44; surveillance capability of, 142–
44; training activities and, 126–28;
use of motion pictures of, 48

World War One, 51; concerns about national health during, 81, 215–16n7;
influenza pandemic and, 55–56,
81, 125, 139–40, 144; promotion of
patriotism during, 209nn30–31;
troop health films in, 55; U.S. Public Health Service films during, 55;
venereal disease and, 56–57, 208n25,
210n39, 215–16n7

World War Two, 51; anti-Asian xenophobia during, 21–22, 193–94, 219n45;
creation of Centers for Disease
Control and Prevention (CDC) and,
124–25; epidemiological mapping
during, 127; military training films
in, 33, 57, 135–38, 208n25, 210n39;
national health focus during, 81, 124–
25, 215–16n7; origins of world health
discourse and, 53, 69–70, 124–26;
sexualized transmission of disease
during, 59–66

X Files, The (TV series), 176

Yoshimoto, Mitsuhiro, 192

KIRSTEN OSTHERR is an assistant professor in the Department of English at Rice University.

LIBRARY OF CONGRESS CATALOGING-IN-PUBLICATION DATA
Ostherr, Kirsten, 1970–
Cinematic prophylaxis : globalization and contagion in the
discourse of world health / Kirsten Ostherr.
p. cm.
Includes bibliographical references and index.
ISBN 0-8223-3635-9 (cloth : alk. paper)
ISBN 0-8223-3648-0 (pbk. : alk. paper)
1. Diseases in motion pictures. 2. Science fiction films—History
and criticism. I. Title.
[DNLM: 1. Disease Outbreaks—prevention & control. 2. Health
Promotion—methods. 3. Attitude to Health. 4. Motion Pictures.
5. Medicine in Art. 6. Internationality. WA 105 O85c 2005]
PN1995.9.D56O88 2006
791.43'6561—dc22   2005011686